Robert Schindele – **Superbiomin®**

Robert Schindele

Superbiomin®

The Superbiomin with its 26 Mineral Elements

for

Human Beings, Animals and Nature

W. ENNSTHALER-VERLAG, A-4402 STEYR

2nd Edition 1993

ISBN 3 85068 285 4

Set, printed and published by Wilhelm Ennsthaler, A-4402 Steyr

TABLE OF CONTENTS

Preface

When in spring 1981 my caterpillar-driver, on the occasion of the construction of a forest road in one of my forest enterprises in the surroundings of Melk in Lower Austria cut twice a volcanic cone of a rather soft, brittle material which emerged from a breach in the earth's crust and was surrounded by very hard paragneiss, I did not anticipate the consequences that were to follow in the future.

On the occasion of an inspection of the location line under construction of this forest road, the project manager Oberforstrat Dipl. Ing. Brandstätter of the Niederösterreichische Landwirtschaftskammer (Chamber of Agriculture of Lower Austria) and Oberforstrat Dipl. Ing. Hans Schoder of the Bezirksbauernkammer Melk suggested, in order to save money, to use this material for the substructure and the ballast of the forest road.

This was done. At the beginning of July 1981, it was very hot at that time, more than six thousend cubic metres were embarked on the location line which was in raw state and graded with my caterpillar. Because of the great heat and the rubbing off of the tyres of the heavy lorrys, a lot of dust was produced.

The dust penetrated 50 meters and more into the woods and covered the ground with a closed layer.

We could also observe another phenomenon.

The chains of the caterpillar became longer and longer every day and we had to take out a link, because the chain could not be tightened any more. My driver, a man with 40 years of work experience said: „I have never had such an experience!" Now we know why this had happened.

Examinations with a polarizing microscope and a roentgen microscope revealed that this is a mineral deposit that has not been found anywhere else in the world and consists of 30% alkali feldspar, 20–30% plagioclase, 20–30% quartz, 15–20% biotite, 5–10% disthene, garnet, silimanite, ore, zircon and rutile.

The 26 mineral elements found up to now have a retrograde transformation of the atomic crystal lattice with transitory metals and retrogression to alkali feldspar.

Because of its containing about 5 % of iron and the trace element cobalt, which is the best magnet, the minerals become highly magnetic by friction. The molecules of the chain links of the caterpillar and of the bolts place themselves at the friction surface in the same direction; the transformation of the atomic crystal lattice also takes place. Even the hardest steel dissolves, layer by layer.

Now back to the road construction.

A few days after the construction of the forest road had been completed, heavy rain fell; the layer of dust disappeared.

At one of the loading points of the minerals a fir tree grows which is about 50 years old. At the time of the ballasting it was yellow and dying and had already been marked for felling. This fir tree should be felled, when the forest was to be thinned out mid-August 1981.

When this was about to be done, one of my forestry workers said: „Why shall we fell this fir tree at the roadside? It is still very green and if we fell it, we would have a big hole in the forest stand."

I went to examin the situation and was extremely surprised, because the tree was dark green und has been prospering well. It had since then developed healthy needles for seven years. I knew immediately that the minerals had caused this change. For several years I just observed and in 1985 I decided to inform the press.

First a well-known scientist examined the place of discovery. He took up a piece of the mineral and said: „This has to work; you can see the potassium with the naked eye, as well as garnets!" He had the material analyzed and sent his first report about this to the Austrian Ministry of Science, for the attention of Ministerialrat Dipl. Ing. Dr. Persey.

Only a few days later Dr. Maria Felsenreich from Gänserndorf arranged a press conference in the „Presseclub Concordia", where I could talk about my observations.

The scientist Dr. Gernot Gräfe explained to the press why the trees recovered again.

In September 1985 the place of discovery of the minerals and the adjacent woods were introduced to the public in the presence of representatives of the Austrian radio and television station (ORF) and high-level polititians. There was a live transmission in the radio;

and while we still were sitting in a restaurant in Emmersdorf discussing this with scientists, the first television broadcast was transmitted in the programme „Österreichbild".

The Austrian radio and television station ORF have informed our people fast and correctly in many broadcasts.

I would like to take this opportunity to express to the ladies and gentlemen in charge my commendation, appreciation and thanks.

This applies also to the many reporters, redactors and employees of the international press, to the many editors of magazins and pictorials, as well as to the radio and television organizations.

Actually only a few days later it was reported worldwide that I had discovered a remedy against the dying of the woods.

Many experiments have shown that well-nourished trees can cope with the stress of the enviroment and that according to the present level of research and with a bit of good will, man can reduce this stress situation during the next decades.

In September 1985 it was clear to me that I would have constructed my own factory for fine grinding of the minerals.

For the time being I had ground a few tons by a factory located nearby. After I had analysed my first own mineral flour, I started to study all the scientific literature I could get hold of, and I decided then to eat a small quantity of these minerals myself.

I thought, if this is good for my trees it should help me too.

After a severe **meat poisoning**, I had for many years strong, painful colics, a very high **uric acid level**, 7,6–7,8; consequences of this high **value of uric acid** were **gout** and a constant festering **tonsilitis**. Only a few hours after I had swallowed the first teaspoon of minerals mixed with water, I had violent eructations. The same day the pressure in the stomach region disappeared. The next day I decided to double the dose. On that the winds were discharged rapidly. After three days I was freed from a ten-year-old sickness. Three weeks later my **gout** had disappeared and the **blood pressure** had dropped from 100/180 to 85/145!

A few weeks later the **tonsilitis** troubles were gone and my snow-white **hair** got some black strands. Meanwhile it has partly turned black again. I then had a **blood test** made, which showed completely normal values. Now I may drink again alcohol and coffee as much as I want; nothing changes. But I must add, that I have been swallowing my minerals every day since 1985.

In March 1986 a long article was published about this in the respectable newspaper „Die Welt". At the same time the „Hessische Rundfunk" and „Radio Luxembourg" reported about it.

Within only a few weeks, this news had gone around the world. Even the Japanese television reported about this.

Every day 1000 to 2000 letters arrived, a flood that could not be coped with. During a broadcast of the Austrian radio called „Wir am Mittwoch" the commentator Mr. Hademar Bankhofer showed to the viewers 10000 letters which had reached the television station within only a few weeks, all asked for my address.

On some days queues of cars of up to one kilometer with customers waited in front of my factory. The telephone rang from 4 am until 11 pm.

One could foresee that taking „Superbiomin" was **not** approved by everybody. Thank goodness the critical attacks could be unbiassed and technically invalidated.

But there were also more agreeable things. In September 1986 „Superbiomin" was exhibited at the Viennese fair „Wiener Messe". After the fair the products exhibited by the Inventors' Association were rated. On this occasion the President of the Inventors' Association said the following: „And today's highlight, „Superbiomin" is awarded the gold medal." He added: „Up to now no inventor or discoverer succeeded to become famous worldwide and to sell worldwide in such a short time."

I had to give a lecture of half an hour and I got more applause than all the other inventors together.

On Saturday, 12 December 1987, a programme about „Superbiomin" was transmitted in the Austrian radio (Ö3) at 3 pm. Ing. Stanislaus Krumpholc was interviewed by telephone. Nineteen years ago he had come to Austria as a refugee, and from his working in a uranium mine he had **antinotoxemia.** He also suffered from **myelopathy**, his hands **trembled** and he had a strong **itching** all over his body. When he heard about „Superbiomin" he came to see us just for fun and swallowed it just like hundreds of thousands other people. Only a few days later, the **tremulation** disappeared as well as all the other damages. Now I know why this had happened. By the retrograde transformation of the atomic lattice of „Superbiomin" it influences the smallest, highly vibrating, and therefore radiant particles of the radioactive precipitation, changes also there the atomic lattice and so intercepts the vibration (radiation).

This is a natural process which will gain importance for the next atomic catastrophe.

The Future or the Destruction of Mankind Lies in the Fertilization of the Soil

Now, a few years after the discovery of the meanwhile world-famous mineral occurrence „Superbiomin", its utilization in agriculture and forestry, by **man** and **animals**, and the many letters I received on the mentioned subjects by my customers and by numerous scientists from many countries, as well as my own experience, I could furnish the proof that for a long time the cause for the **sickliness** of man, animal und plant is the insufficient supply of the soil with minerals and trace elements and the wrong application of some of the fertilizers and the resulting acid rain which causes the death of the soil bacteria and the **mycorrhiza** (symbiosis between roots, seed plants und funghi).

To my horror I have repeatedly observe that many farmers scatter burnt lime on their fields. Thus they kill many soil bacteria and all the micro-organisms und funghi, which are essential for the formation of humus and the mineralization. The liming of the soil should only be done with unslaked, pulverized calcium carbonate, or, preferrably, with dolomite, which contains a lot of magnesium. Magnesium absorbs the acid in the soil and increases the pH-value. Magnesium is the central atom of the chlorophyll molecule, which is absolutely necessary for the reception of carbon. About 15 to 20% of the magnesium content are absorbed by the chlorophyll molecule and thus activate many enzymes (carbohydrate metabolism) and facilitate the reception and the transport of phosphates. Deficiency of magnesium causes by plants chlorosis. The leafs of the trees turn yellow und fall off prematurely, the fruit of the fruit trees do not ripen fully, get tough and do not taste any more the way they should. Magnesium is responsible for the chlorophyll and the photosynthesis of the sunlight.

The soil bacteria which should be sufficiently available in the healthy soil secrete various acids and thus dissolve the minerals and metals of the soil, as far as they are there at all. Large areas of the earth have too little minerals. In the alps (except in areas with clay and loam deposits) there is hardly any potassium, no silicic acid, no iron und many important trace elements exist only in insufficient quantities. This is the area, where most of the larch trees grow. The larch trees secrete hydrochloric acid at the roots with which it dissolves parts of the limestone rock and therefore can nourish itself also in barren regions.

The soil bacteria eat the dissolved minerals and trace elements, digest them and excrete them in the form of ions (smallest fractions split off atoms by absorbing or releasing an electron). These ions can be absorbed by the plants and the trees and are transmitted by means of the natural food-chain to the animals and man. If some mineral elements are missing also the food-chain is disturbed which results in deficiency symptoms. The withered soil bacteria serve the plants as organic food. The funghis, on the other hand, form with the roots of the plants and trees and with the bacteria a symbiosis. The roots of the plants secrete nutrive substances (mainly glucose), which serve funghis and bacteria as nourishment. These, on the other hand, give to the plants salts and minerals they can absorbe, which serve not only as nutrients, but also to build defensive substances against harmful funghis and various diseases. Well-nourished plants and trees can very well distinguish between useful and harmful funghis. They also have a well functioning communication system, by means of which they can communicate at long distances, which enables them e.g., if they are parasitized by pests, to build defensive substances in good time. This phenomenon is described in the book of the personally known American **authors Christopher Bird and Peter Tompkin, of the bestseller „Das geheime Leben der Pflanzen**, Pflanzen als Lebewesen mit Charakter und Seele und ihre Reaktionen in den physischen und emotionellen Beziehungen zum Menschen", published by Fischer Verlag in Frankfurt/Main. In this book scientists of the whole world, who worked in this field of research, are listed with their names und addresses, have exactly described this phenomenon. I can only recommend to everybody to read this book. One thing is clear, the communication is made by means of odiferous substances, partly with an up to now undiscovered wavelength.

Waves actually play an important role in all spheres of life.

All life, whether of the human being, the animal or the plant, depends on audible and even more on inaudible waves in the ultrasonic sphere up to milliards of vibrations per second, or on the infrasonic waves, one vibration per second or less. Vibrations are at the same time radiation. Vibrations in the highest sphere are felt as warmth. All living creatures, plants, trees, animals or human beings possess a measurable active radiation called aura. Trained scientists can identify an injured tree without looking at its treetop just by its weakened aura. In the book of Christopher Bird it is described how trees und plants that are immersed with warbling of birds und good music, grow much faster than others. Russian scientists found out, that using activated water produces 30 % more vegetation. The same phenomenon was proved through experiments by the late, famous head forester Schauberger. The easiest way to activate water is to atomize it under high pressure (8 to 10 bars). But, on the other hand, certain vibrations (radiations) can be harmful. Trees that stand on water veins (water veins are already measurable with appropriate instruments) become stunted, they turn away from the water vein, just as if they wanted to escape. Crossed water veins cause after years or decades, depending on the condition of the human being or the animal, inevitably cancer. The damaging frequency of this radiation paralyzes the cell membrane, where the cause of all illness lies. Sensitive people may cause severe car accidents, when driving over a water vein and involuntarily jerk the steering wheel violently. The radiation of high-tension transmission lines are also very harmful. Bee colonies staying under them, lose their interest in gathering honey, get agressive and finally they stab oneanother to death. The radiation of all electric devices, radio and television, especially of the transmitters, have bad consequences on our nervous system. One of the reasons for the dying of the woods are electromagnetic waves. In edition no. 102 of the „Stuttgarter Holzzentralblatt" dated 26 August 1987 it says: „Was the research on the dying of the woods mislead?" The primary cause for the dying of the woods is the environmental pollution by microwaves.

In order to acquaint you with these findings, I cite below the article mentioned.

Extract from article of the „Holzzentralblatt", Stuttgart, 26. August 1987

Possibilities to Put an End to the Dying of the Woods

The military radar was one of the first causes of the dying of the woods in our region between East and West. In the GDR it is mainly the Sowjet radar that „cuts off" the woods on the crest of the Erz Mountain. In the upper Black Forest the French radar installations on the left bank of the Rhine, are the malefactors.

In the Rhön and the Franconian Forest are, in addition to the military radar, powerful civil transmitting stations directed towards the GDR. In the Alps the rock walls function like mirrors and produce microwaves, which normally are absorbed by the well-wooded slopes of the Mittelgebirge. By means of these reflections, microwaves also enter woods, where there are no high-tension transmitting stations in the field of vision.

With a bit of good will on the part of the army, one could stop the mischief in peacetime, to operate the radar installations nearly 24 hours a day. It would be sufficient to check the radar installations in the same intervals as the civil or air raid protection sirens. The personnel could be trained in desert regions far from civilization. Apart from that, the military directional transmitters and radar installations should be included in the missiles and disarmament negotiations. Both, the East und the West could appreciate that thus one of the greatest causers of the dying of the woods could be eliminated.

Now back again to fertilization, in particular to dunging with liquid manure. If scattered too early, the soil gets back not only nitrogen, potassium and phosphates, but also harmful putrefactive bacteria get into the soil, which cannot be broken down fast enough, which means, that they are absorbed by the plants, when still alive, and thus get through the food-chain (salads etc.) into our digestive tract. The liquid manure should remain long enough in the pits and stone, containing a lot of minerals and reduced to powder, should be added again and again. With these minerals other bacteria and funghi develop, which then break down the putrefactive bacteria and remove the bad smell. The same applies to stable manure. If scattered well putrified and decomposed, it does not harm, if scattered too early, it poisens the soil and the drinking water. It hardly contributes to humification, because the excrements of animals are nutrient-poor. Vegetables that were manured only with stable manure or with fresh liquid manure can be harmful for infants, since the existing and not so quickly degradable toxic substances indole, skatole, putrescine and toxic phenols lead to hypochrome anaemia.

Too much fertilization with nitrogen can also cause poisoning of the drinking water. The nitrogen fertilizer not used quickly by the plants, converts to nitrate and poisons our drinking water. This is one of the greatest threats to mankind, because with the many exhaust gases of the cars, nitrogen oxide gets into the soil, i.e. ca. 100 kg pure nitrogen per hectare (100000 m^2) per year!

The former director of the Bundesanstalt für Qualitätsforschung (Federal Agency for Quality Control) in Gneisenheim, FRG, Prof. Schuphan, announced the following research results: „Nitrogen fertilizers – nitrates – make our food plants more susceptible to diseases and to parasitisation. The high content of nitrogen reduces the vitamins and mineral elements of the plant." When he was still alive, Prof. Schuphan often pointed out, that during the past years symptoms of poisoning (cyanosis) of the babies were observed to a life threatening extent, which has been caused by too high amounts of nitrite in spinach and kohlrabi. On 24 February 1987 the „Kronen Zeitung" reported on page 8 about wide-spread deaths of roe deers, who had catcn rape. The digestive organs and the brain of the animals were damaged. The haemoglobin transformed to methaemoglobin. The oxygen supply of the heart and the brain was blocked. The animals became blind, deaph and lost their olfactory sense and therefore died a miserable death.

The question arises now, could the same happen to us, when we eat vegetables. In the countries of the European Community the content of nitrate in drinking water should not exceed 90 mg/liter. In shallow water veins values of more than 500 mg/liter were reported.

When fertilizing with nitrogen, one should be aware of the fact that soil bacteria exist which can bind nitrogen with the help of cobalt up to an amount of 60 kg/ha per year and can reduce fertilizing cost. This anaerobic Clostridium-Bacterium lives in acid soils with a pH-value of up to 4.5. Moreover, nitrogen is produced by nodule bacteria, the Rhizobia. But they can only live in a symbiosis with the leguminosae. Nitrogen is also produced by blue-green algaes and green algaes. It is assumed that the mycorrhiza, funghis living in a symbiosis with the roots, are able to produce nitrogen. Nitrogen is sufficiently available in the air, 8 tons per m^2 ground space. But, fortunately, the plants are not able to absorb anything of this surplus. This is a wise measure of nature which makes it possible for us to live.

In the technical part of the „Bauernbündler" of Lower Austria dated 26 February 1987, I just read a very interesting article with the title „Lime nitrogen: Purposeful application in the modern plant breeding brings many advantages." The only advantage I realize is that the nitrogen is given off slowly. The author of the article made some serious mistakes. He describes its corrosive, weed controling effect. He saves – or reduces – in many cases the application of chemical herbicides. Again burnt lime which kills the soil bacteria is used as a carrier. With three to four dt/ha lime nitrogen scattered before the beginning of the vegetation, liver flukes and other parasites of pastures are combatted. Lime nitrogen improves the composition of the standing crop. Weeds like chickweed, speedwell and especially **dandelion** can be combatted effectively.

I am greatly astonished to realize how ignorant are (bad the education is at) the universities, otherwise such severe mistakes may not have happened. The author fails to see that chickenweed, speedwell and dandelion are medical herbs that animals need as much as human beings. Dandelion is a food speciality and takes effect very successfully against hepatopathy. The only good posibility to fertilize the soil and keep alive the soil organisms, while increasing at the same time the nutrient content to improve food plants, is to use the mineral powder to which non-corrosive fertilizer customary in trade is added.

The silicon (silic acid) is of utmost importance for all living creatures. The supporting structure of the cells consists of silicic acid crystals. Silicic acid crystals (quartz) emit waves which serve to stimulate the cell membranes. If the cell membranes do not function, harmful virusses can enter the cells, where they reproduce themselves, and some kinds of virus can attack the desoxyribonucleic acid that is accummulated in the chromosomes. Considering that the number of chromosomes, 42 or 43, already decides, if a male or a female comes into being, and with a mutation (44 chromosomes) a mentally deficient human being suffering from debility develops, one may find here the cause for the scourage of mankind, cancer. Since the cells live for about 8 months and continuously new cells are produced, uncontrolable excrescences, tumours must develop, if the genes are damaged.

The **German food chemist Dr. Mang from Frankfort on the Main wrote on this subject the following: The Original Schindele's mineral cure** consists of pulverized natural rock flow, with a high content of **silicic acid**, aluminium, potassium, iron, magnesium, as well as numerous trace elements. The mineral elements are, just like the protein, fat and carbohydrates, considerably involved in the course of the life process, by helping to create the physical and chemical conditions for the functioning of the cells. Mineral elements influence growth and the haemopoiesis and are strongly connected with the anabolism of hormons, vitamins and **enzymes**. They are very important elements of the **bones, teeth** and special tissues. Since they are continuously exchanged and lost, they have to be given to the body regularly. Deficiency of mineral elements over long periods are for human beings the cause of deficiency diseases. If one takes regularly the original Schindele's mineral cure, the organism receives sufficient mineral elements, therefore a deficiency of mineral elements can be excluded. The **orginal Schindele's mineral cure** is to be considered a **„real food"** which is virtually a natural substance without toxic substances.

For the functioning of the cells, sufficient oxygen supply is certainly necessary. Iron and potassium serve best as transporter of the oxygen (the center of the blood pigment, the haemoglobin, consists of iron ions). Potassium can be accumulated in the body only for eight hours, and therefore has to be supplied by the food, if this is not possible, then by taking minerals. **Hypertension** can be normalized with potassium and magnesium. Silicic acid, this should be added, is for human beings and animals essential for the structure of the **sinews, eyes, the ear conches**, as well as for the **nails**, claws or cloven hoofs. Silicic acid (silicon) strengthens the structure of the cells of plants and trees. They get more elastic and therefore cannot easily be broken by the wind. The grain does not so easily get to the lying position that is dreaded so much.

Now back again to potassium. This base, easily soluble metal is, in combination with oxygen (K_20),involved in the functions of the cell membrane and the sensitive process of the enzyme activities, i.e. potassium is involved in the action potential of at least 40 hormones and promotes the somatic setup of energy releasing substances in the cellular structure. Human beings have up to 98 % of the potassium intracellularly in the cell sap, mainly in the muscular tissue. The rest is bound to glycogen or phosphates. Potassium is rapidly absorbed from the chyme in the upper part of the small intestine, into the blood circulation. It completes its task then, and since the body does not have the capability to accumulate potassium, 95 % are quickly excreted by the kidneys, the faeces and the swet. Every cell needs potassium for its biological growth and its optimal reactivity. Potassium is only active, if natrium is available as opponent. This important biological correlation between potassium and natrium is of great importance for the undisturbed transport of the vehicles of energy to the cells, this is especially true for nerve fibres and muscular functions.

Within the cell concentration of natrium is normally low, while the concentration of potassium is high. Outside of the cell the situation is just the other way round. Potassium and natrium are two vital mineral elements which are essential for the regulation and the maintenance of the normal blood pressure. Potassium and natrium complement each other. Potassium activates the elimination of water, natrium binds water in the body. Potassium is a part of every cell in the human body. During each cell activity, the intracellular potassium is exchanged through the cell membrane with natrium inits immediate surrounding. Potassium controls the pressure and the swelling in the cellular tissue. The cell can hold potassium only with the help of magnesium. This exchange of electrically charged ions is the basis for the activity of the nerves and the muscular functions. For the conductivity of the nervous system, calcium ions are necessary. The potassium activates the regular beat of the heart and influences the formation of enzymatic systems and makes available and accumulates energy. It supports the regular transmission of nerve impulses. Lack of potassium in the **cardiac muscle** can cause sudden **death by cardiac failure, disturbances of the cardiac rhythm** reduced and irregular **pulse**, change the ECG and cause long-term damages. Lack of potassium causes colics, constipation and lack of apetite. It paralyzes the biological peristaltic movement and causes further paralysis that can spread from the neck along the body. Lack of potassium causes muscular weakness, general fatigue and decline in performance. It causes sudden blood sugar fall. For plants and trees potassium is vital for the protective wax layer on leafs and needles. If the protective wax layer on leafs and needles is not strong enough, pollutants can penetrate quickly and start their destructive activities.

Another important mineral is calcium.

Its most important function for man and animal is the construction of the **bones** and the **teeth**. But for this, there has to be the right ratio of phosphate, otherwise it results in the dreaded **brittleness of the bones**. Both, calcium as well as phosphates are stored in the bone tissue and can be used for other bodily functions. Therefore they too have to be constantly replaced. Extremely important for soil bacteria as well as for plants, human beings and animals are the trace elements manganese, copper, zinc, cobalt, molybdenum, boron, chromium, nickel, vanadium, selenium, arsenic etc. These metals are in a special correlation to oneanother and help to build up a lot of the enzymes. To be able to function well, the organisms need only small quantities of these metals. If they are partly or completely missing, serious deficiency symptoms are the consequence. The infertility of animals and probably also of the human beings is caused by the lack of copper.

Iron serves to transport the oxygen to the cells, especially to the **cardiac muscles** and to the **brain**. It is known that a cardiac arrest of only 10 minutes already causes severe brain damages, due to the lack of oxygen. Lack of iron also causes disturbances of the lipid metabolism and lack of oxygen which the cells need for the burning and the production of energy. Iron tablets or minerals containing iron and vitamin E tablets which support the sexual potency, should be taken in an interval of two hours; if taken together, they cause sickness, the consequence of a shock.

Also plants absolutely need iron for their metabolism and the photosynthesis. Plants that do not get enough iron, turn yellow (green sickness, chlorosis). Especially much iron is needed by children and by women during their **menstruation** or during **pregnancy**.

The trace elements among the metals are absolutely the most important regulators for the production of enzymes, and because of their correlation to one another they always should be taken together, since one alone can get toxic (poisonous).

This regulatory mechanism stems from the fact, that all life comes from the sea, and that the sea water, as the basis for all living creatures (human being, animal, plant), contains all mineral elements.

Only natrium which was constantly washed in from the land, increased constantly, since it cannot evaporate.

One of the most important regulating metals for human beings, animals and plants is chromium. In 1935 the scientists Scharrer and Schopp made experiments with corn cereal, whereby chromium was added to soil with little chromium and they found out that it had a positive effect on the growth and the compositon of the plants.

Only fourvalent to sixvalent chromium can turn toxic. It changes in the soil rapidly back to the vital Chrom III. This should be taken into consideration, if sewage sludge containing chromium is distributed on the soil! The distribution should take place after the vegetative period. The change has taken place before the next vegetative period starts. The plant takes from the soil only what it needs!

For the human being and the animal chromium is essential for the fat metabolism and the glucose metabolism.

Since by the gastric acid only a small part is dissolved and by the intestinal flora again another small part, the grown-up person needs about 2 mg per day, animals ca. 3 mg per 100 g body weight.

If the necessary quantities of chromium are missing, this causes inevitably arteriosclerosis of the **coronary vessels** and **diabetes**. This is one of the greatest crimes of all against the health of man and animal. The knowledge in research is so extensive that **diabetes** should not exist at all any more.

The same applies to many other severe diseases.

Below, I would like to draw the attention to other metals!

Cobalt, a heavy, hard metal, forms with manganese the „mantle" of vitamin B_{12} in four enzymes.

If cobalt is missing – then no nucleic acid synthesis can take place and **anaemia** is the consequence. If manganese is missing, no **ureopoiesis** takes place, and the citric acid cycle is blocked! If zinc is missing, **muscular poisoning**, alcoholic poisoning, acidosis and the stop of the protein synthesis will happen. Without nickel no **urea splitting** can take place. Lack of zinc causes the stop of the secretion of the digestive ferments. Aluminium is also necessary for the digestion. Molybdenum is very important for the memory. If it is missing, disturbances of the purine oxidation and the fatty acid formation from carbohydrates take place.

We even need, in small quantities, for the function of our eyes, the poison arsenic, which is latal, if taken in greater quantities. We find sufficient quantities of arsenic in the onion. Famous doctors of ancient times (e.g. Paracelsus) said: „It always depends on the quantity, if it helps or not!"

So it may shock some people to learn that we also need, in very small quantities, strontium, barium, silver, lead, cadmium, rubidium, antimony, sulfur, fluorine and titanium and many other elements, to ensure that all our body functions can be maintained at all.

I would like to point out, that minerals that are meant for human consumption, have to be examined scientifically very carefully, i.e. as to their solubility in gastric acid, because thus the quantity, that we have available during the digestive process of two days, can be determined exactly. Also the interchange of electrons and the electrical conductivity have to be as high as possible!

The edible deposits I discovered that have not been discovered anywhere else in the world, consist of alkali feldspar, plagioclase, quartz, biotite, disthene, garnet, silimanite, ore, zircon and rutile. It possesses a retrograde transformation of the atomic lattice with a retrogression to alkali feldspar with transitory metals. Because of this procedure it produces current which makes it easy to detect falsification very easily with the help of measuring instruments, before the chemical analysis is made.

A thousands of years old knowledge from the aristocracy reports that precious stones should be worn not because of their value, but, depending on the colour of the stones, to stimulate the different organs by the respective waves.

But there exist also minus pole deposits. These are absolutely unsuited for man, animals and plants.

For my own experience, and from the many letters of my clients who eat my **mineral flour „Superbiomin"**®, diseases disappear that, up to now, were considered incurable. After only a few weeks, **diabetic values** of 280 and more, are reduced to 80–90, **gout** disappears, the **blood pressure** and all other values balance out to normal, the **values of uric acid** increase for a short period (dissolution of sediments) and then drop again quickly. The faeces turn black for a few months, later get normal again.

But if one stops taking the minerals for several weeks, all complaints come back again. By this fact, I could prove that the reason for at least 90% of all diseases of human beings, animals and plants are caused by the lack of mineral elements in our food, and therefore by the lack of mineral elements and by the lack of the respective bacteria. In order to be able to determine these deficiencies, the soil samples have to be examined as to their content of minerals, as well as to their content of microorganism and mykorrhiza (funghis). Already in 1940, when the soil conditions were much better than today, the Swiss medical doctor, Dr. Zimmermann who became famous by his book „Steine geben Brot", wrote the following: „Our food does no longer deserve to be called food, we only fill our stomach." He also suggested that the appropriate minerals should be eaten, as has been done by old civilized nations already thousands of years ago. He wrote on this subject: *„The digestive tract of the human being is of vegetable nature. Give from now on stones to the human being e.g. in form of finely ground* *stone flour, tiny quantities are dissolved, just like it is done by the plant. The rest leaves the body without doing any harm." (Sand cleans the stomach, a proverb says). Therefore a human being can very well eat 100 grams of stone powder, he or she will not endure any bad effects. Indeed, vitamins that we take as restorative roborant, are ineffective without trace elements as co-factor.*

The **formation of stones** in the **kidney** and in the **bile** cannot happen, since the formation of stones is caused by the lack of mineral elements.

Only if an agriculture all fields and meadows are constantly fertilized with all the necessary minerals (which is only possible with stone flours containing a lot of silicon which contains all the necessary elements) we will again have healthy food, healthy animals and healthy human beings, and we need no longer swallow minerals as a complement to the food.

I want to draw your attention to some other dangers that threaten us.

One of them is the lack of oxygen, up to now unnoticed, which will emerge one day, due to the hundreds of millions of cars, large thermic firing installations and forest fires etc. It is certainly known that 60% of our oxygen is produced by the plankton in the seas, 40% by the woods and the plants. Chemical poisons that are used in the industry and in agriculture are let into the sea as waste waters and kill a lot of plankton. A second threat arises from the pollution of oil through drilling towers and ships. Already an extremely thin film of oil that covers already huge areas of the sea, is sufficient to reflect the sunlight, just like a mirror. No more photosynthesis takes place, the plankton is reduced by the natural consumption by the sea animals, the production of oxygen will be reduced, due to the dying of the woods, the building up of large areas and the increase of desert regions. This is a vicious circle to which there is no escape. Without oxygen no combustition engine runs. The car industry will have to switch to electric cars. The energy production will have to be effected by other energy ressources, by water (also tidal power) and wind, sun and the temperature of the interior of the earth. Another very great danger is the ozon in the air that is produced by photo oxidation of the exhaust gases. The ozon is the main cause for the dying of the woods. It has a corrode effect on the needles and the leafs, kills the soil organisms, that live in the upper layer of humus and that are responsible for splitting up the minerals, including the important penicillin producing mucedines, as well as all other funghis. Ozon damages our respiration organs and quickly affects all metals except gold, plantinum and iridium, as well as all buildings.

It will be even worse with the woods. Most foresters who go through the woods blindly, did not yet realize that the rootstocks of all trees that are older than 50 years, and that are thinner than a finger, are already dead or rotten.

Since most of the nutric substances and most of the water are taken up by these rootstocks, our trees must starve and die of thirst, because the fine rootstocks are missing. It is no longer possible to save most of the woods, because of lack of money. It would be possible to save the woods of an age of up to 50 years with stone flours, containing a lot of silicate and minerals. But again, there is not enough money. And for most forest enterprises, there will be less and less money available. Since we have had a series of dry years, our trees are still embedded in the hard and dry soil. But watch out, if a wet year comes. The slightest wind will knock down whole regions, the price for wood will decay completely, the enourmous quantites turning up simultaneously will no longer be coped with and sold. The many insect pests will mulitply uncontrolably and kill the younger, still standing forest crops. In the alps whole regions will become uninhabitable, due to avalanches of snow and mudflows, the tourism will therefore be reduced considerably, the income from foreign exchange will decrease, the people living in these areas will have to leave and will push into the deteriorating employment market and no longer be able to find work. It will become even worse, if, because of the decay of the price for wood which will come with absolute certainty, numerous mountain peasants who live a great deal or entirely on the profits of the wood will be ruined and cannot find work anywhere. Here lies the basis for the next revolution that we cannot be spared. The anger of the people is always directed against the respective ruling class. I would not want to be a politician then.

Robert Schindele

The Application of „Superbiomin"

How to Apply „Superbiomin"

1 teaspoon of „Superbiomin" in the morning o r in the evening, drink thereafter a lot of water, or even better, milk, or any other liquid.

The same way „Superbiomin" can be taken in the morning a n d in the evening.

„Superbiomin" can be dissolved in the above-mentioned quantities in water, milk or in other liquids and then drunk.

„Superbiomin" as Skin Cream

„Superbiomin" can be made into an effective skin cream by mixing well „Superbiomin" with a skin cream available on the market, in a ratio of 1:1. This takes especially good effect against the formation of wrinkles in the face.

Face Pack with „Superbiomin"

A wonder drug against wrinkled skin.

Ingredients: 1 tablespoon „Superbiomin"
1 teaspoon honey
1 yolk

All ingredients are mixed well in a cup until the mixture is easy to spread. This face pack is applied onto the well cleaned face and the neck. Let it work on the skin for 10–20 minutes, then wash off with a lot of cold water. This mask can be repeated 1–2 times a week.

„Superbiomin" as an Admixture to the Bath

Dissolve 500 g „Superbiomin" in ca.5 l of water (70°C maximum). This admixture to the bath is added to the bath water. While bathing the bath water should be stirred several times. The bathing time should be ca. 1/2 hours.

„Superbiomin" baths take effect against **rheumatic pains** and **fatigue**, regenerate the body and improve the general well-being. „Superbiomin" baths also lifts the skin.

„Superbiomin" in Bread-Making

1 tablespoon „Superbiomin" is added to 1 kg dough.

Through „Superbiomin" the taste of the bread is improved and the body is supplied with additional mineral elements.

„Superbiomin" can also be added, when baking cakes and gateaus.

„Superbiomin" for Animals

10 g „Superbiomin" per day per 70 kg live weight.

By adding „Superbiomin" to the food the fitness of riding horses and other animals is stimulated.

„Superbiomin" for Flowers

Flowers too like „Superbiomin".

2 x per year spread one heaped teaspoon „Superbiomin" over the garden mould, add lots of water.

Test Reports

***University Professor E. K.-L. from Switzerland,* full professor of the National Cooperating University of America N. C., writes on 7 August 1986:**

Dear Mr. SCHINDELE,

For four months we have been employing, in addition to our system and method – „athermic pulsating electronic magnetic high frequency fields and waves – DIAPULE – generator pulsators" – as a supplement – the high-grade bio-minerals. The patients come to our house only after all pharmacon programmes had been employed and had not brought the expected results.

The NASA-technique – which has been employed by us successfully since 1973 – now brings a faster regeneration, e.g. with reduced formation of callus after fractures, and they now stay here for a time in this situation that has been reduced by 60%.

After a cardiac infarct, we notice, within a few days, a faster, better circulation of the blood of the arterial blood circulation and a very fast strengthening of the cardiac muscle. The patient is freed from the pain on pressure within only a few days, because the biochemical liquid which washes around the cardiac muscle, is influenced very positively by the bio-mineral elements. The blood pressure is also regulated rapidly. The statement: With acute and chronical, inflamed processes of the softparts and with joint diseases, i.e. of the rheumatic formenkreis, we reach with additional doses of the bio-minerals from the Haus SCHINDELE faster reduction of the pain and faster movability of the joints. In severe cases of deformed polyarthritis, we get faster to the pharmaca maintenance dose, until the way has been reached to a longer stagnation. We all know that the rheumatic formenkreis is a hereditary defect and therefore cannot be cured, but life gets more worth living for people of this group..., merely biologically formed. Certainly, this group of patients has to goback to the appartus time after time, but the severe relapsing quota do not exist any more.

For decades we have known that illnesses of human beings and animals, are due to the reduction of mineral elements in the liver and metabolism of the cells, and therefore to the deformed crystals on the cell membrane – where all illnesses lie – which cannot be washed away properly by the kidney.

We would recommend to every growing person from childhood, to add consciously to the food bio-minerals as a daily supplement to the food. Thus regulating the mineral level, we would see a healthier generation grow up, and the cost would be reduced to a great extent for the insurances and health insurances.

The soils are overacified, because of thoughtless production of chemicals – and so the mineral elements, in the components offered by the HAUS SCHINDELE, are no longer available.

Now we begin with studies of nervous diseases of different degrees- ... further studies will follow during the next years.

We wish the HAUS SCHINDELE further success.

With best regards

***University Professor E. K.-L. from Switzerland,* full professor of the National Cooperating University of America N. C., wrote on 3 November 1986:**

Confirmation:

Dear Mr. Schindele,

During the past six months of this year 1986, the undersigned made the following observations with the patients of our INSTITUTE.

Your SUPER – BIO – MINERAL is the most useful mineral mixture for the human organism.

With this mixture, the mineral metabolism is again fully compensated.

Already the high content of magnesium in these super-minerals reduces many complaints, like muscle spasms of a light degree in the area of the shoulder and the neck – cramps in the calf – headache caused by sensitivity to noise.

Magnesium produces its full, quick and reliable effect only through the overall combination of the mineral mixture that makes up your super-mineral.

Calcariuria and similar unwanted ossifications are influenced in such a way that a washing off of these undesirable states can be observed. The biological balance could thus be established.

Kidney stones caused by stress are less frequent, when giving this super-mineral.

When treating severe vascular diseases, e.g. varicos ulcer, where repeatedly and ascertainably an amputation had been planned, with bio-electric pulsing magnetic fields and adding your super-mineral, a reduction of the pain was rapidly induced, the blood vessels became more permeable and more elastic.

A lack of these minerals, first of all results in a vasoconstriction and thus a heart attack can be favoured.

So, lack of this well-balanced combination of minerals containing such a high content of magnesium, represent a risk factor for the human heart, since it not only increases sensitivity towards stress, but also the reactivity of the heart and the vascular muscular systems to stress hormons.

In addition to a general tendency towards oversensitivity of the cardiac muscle and, as a consequence, pain in the heart and shooting pains in the heart region, disturbances of the cardiac rhythm and cramps in the heart region also of the smooth musculature – are often the consequences of lack of this valuable mineral mixture.

There are countries on the earth, where nearly no mineral elements of this kind can be found; Thailand, Finland or Canada, where a high morbidity quota of the described illness can be noticed.

The super-minerals from the HAUS SCHINDELE with the anorganic mineral elements like magnesium, are absolutely necessary for the anabolism and for all functions of the human body.

If you want to avoid civilizational diseases or want to avoid them to a great extent, you need not add various kinds of tablets, but should start to change your eating habits. Eat preferably a lot of green and leaf vegetables – well-balanced, food with high nutritious value and add the minerals. There are no contra-indications, since, if you take too high a dose of these minerals, they are discharged by every healthy kidney.

This mineral composition, this can be confirmed by the undersigned, cleans the human body, is restorative, activating and stimulating.

Potassium, calcium, phosphates, zinc, magnesium with the rest trace element water, serve the entire bone growth.

With our system and the method, and the addition, we have with osteoporosis, spongiosa and disturbances of growth, a noticeably shorter way to success than before.

Well, in our Institute, we have had excellent success with the bone growth and the maintenance of the bone metabolism.

This mineral combination copper, manganese, organic nitrogens, again with the trace element water, serves the cleaning of the body fluids.

The mineral elements potassium, calcium and the phosphates that are contained therein, help to cure desmopathy that so often can be observed.

In this mineral combination there is a large portion of iron which serves for the increase of oxygen absorption of the blood – do not be afraid, if the faeces turn black during this cure, this is how iron reacts.

This cure, this is my advice, should be carried out during a period of six weeks in a very exact manner, then six weeks of pause, then repeat it. This cure should be made in autumn and in spring.

This is how you take it: In the morning and in the evening dissolve one slightly heaped teaspoon of minerals in a lot of good water, since the super-mineral swells a bit, slowly add a lot of fresh water, drink slowly.

You can apply it as described above, either as a cure oras an addition to the food, the super-mineral is in any case purely biological and has an absolute degree of fineness.

For your information I would like to add that the magnesium contained therein, has also a share of 2.5% of the structure of the earth's crust.

Thus I have paraphrased truthfully the experiences we have had in our INSTITUE.

waren-test-schweiz

First Organization for Consumer Protection, Switzerland (since 1959).

TEST: Fitness flour („Superbiomin") Berne 29 August 1986

Trade Mark	Tolerance	Effect	Side Effects	Result
Superbiomin	excellent***	good***	none***	excellent

1. Testee female, initials L.K.:

„I took the fitness-flour („Superbiomin") during a longer period and am going to continue to do this in future. Twice a day I take one teaspoon in a liquid. Since then I have had normal discharge of the bowels and much less head ache. This same amount I give to my dog, he belongs to a small race, and I noticed that the wound he had for a long time, now has healed and is dry, and that he feels well."

2. Testee male, initials I.S.:

„For 10 weeks I have been taking the fitness flour („Superbiomin") in yoghurt.
I feel again fit and strong. The greatest part of my hair has turned back to its original brown colour and the psoriasis on my left elbow has nearly disappeared completely. My dog, he belongs to a big race, who gets one table spoon of the fitness flour with his food, seems to feel young again and plays again with other dogs."

waren-test schweiz

Reports on successful application

Mr. Dipl.-Ing. Th. Dieter G. from W./FRG writes:

Unasked, I would like to inform you of the results of my own 7-months personal test of your stone flour „Superbiomin" (Su.).

On 3 June 1986 I personally bought your „Superbiomin" from your factory in Kicking. Since that time, I have been taking 2 teaspoons every day. I am 73 years old, chemical engineer and my last position was ina managerial function at „Deutsche Gasrußwerke" in Dortmund, a subsidiary company of DEGUSSA.

1. My **nervous system** including my **memory** now functions again normally and very well. In 1985, due to a six months lasting very inconvenient **strain** of physical and psychological nature, I experienced for the first time in my life an enormous **feeble condition.** For example, I started to be frightened when driving on the autobahn at a speed of 115 km. Furthermore, when driving through the narrow valleys full of curves of the Ticino, Centovalli, Onsernone, Maggia . . . at a speed of 40–50 km/h – I felt for the first time in my life – sick and dizzy. Now I drive again normally, with a speed of up to 200 km/h and also through narrow, crooked valleys (the Dolomites) – this I tried out in September 1986.

2. At the beginning of the eighties, my **right joint of the thumb** had been destroyed incurably, because of a long during, mechanical **overstrain**; it hurt permanently. Now, with the application of „Superbiomin", the pain has disappeared.

3. My **fitness** and tenacity, mental as well as physical, are due to „Superbiomin" back to normal again and very well.

4. The **decay of the skin and the nails** I have had for 30 years, caused by **psoriasis**, disappeared on my hands and are much better on my feet, due to „Superbiomin".

5. The **sexual behaviour** is back to normal, i.e. according to my age, not more, but also not less!!

To sum up: „Superbiomin" has helped me tremendously. The above was discussed with my doctor. And he too does not see any other cause than your stone flour.

In my opinion „Superbiomin" is no wonder drug, no elixier for eternal youth and sexual potency! But in cases of **deficiencies**, caused by factors like nourishment and overstress, it can improve the individual's constitution and heel!! Every person has to try for himself/herself. To get even understanding people to do this, is, according to my experience, so to say impossible!! It is a mistake to give to people „Superbiomin" as a present. They do not take it.

I would like to thank your for your help to help oneself and wish you a lot of success with testing „Superbiomin" with human beings, animals and plants.

Mr. Josef G. from H./FRG writes:

I promised to report to you about my progress.

In July 1986 I ordered for the first time the stone flour and applied it, because, despite taking medicine, I constantly had **pain in the joints**. Since that time I do not take any more medicine and I no longer have **pain in the joints**. I started with taking a teaspoon twice per day and for the last months only one teaspoon per day and I feel well.

Mr. Karl B. from Sch./FRG writes:

Since June 1986 my wife and I have been taking the stone flour – two teaspoons per day.

My wife is 73 years old. She suffered very much from **decalcification of the bones**, constantly had **backache** and could bend only with effort. Since about two months ago these complaints have disappeared. Because of side effects of the respective medicines my wife did not take any medicines nor did she get injections. We therefore attribute the disappearance of the complaints to her taking the mineral flour.

I am 80 years old and used to suffer from rheumatism in the **knees** and in the **ankle joints**. These complaints have nearly disappeared. My **power of concentration** has improved considerably. Because of side effects, I, too, did not take any medicine, nor did I receive injections. I am convinced that your mineral flour has also on me an excellent effect.

Mr. Franz Ferdinand B. from I./Austria writes:

For several years I have had **saccharometabolic** problems. My empty values were, on the average, between 130–155 mg – despite treatment with insulin. After having taken Biomin regularly for five weeks, the values returned to normal, to 96–120 mg on the average.

Mr. R. W. from Pf./FRG writes:

I hardly can understand how it happened, but I came to „Superbiomin" through the information of one of your representatives.

I have been working as a self-employer in the garage business and – it is hardly possible otherwise – especially nowadays, overloaded with work **(stress)**, up to the limit.

Again and again I consulted medical doctors and pharmacists, from my customers and others, in order to find help and support for my overwrought body and organs (thirteen doctors and four pharmacists). Unfortunately, there was no success at all,or just a short-term improvement.

The information and explanations given by your representative convinced me, expecially the comparison with nature, e.g. a plant that is not fed, does not get nutrive substances, also degenerates to insufficient quality.

Now, after writing about my situation before I started to take „Superbiomin", an account of the reactions of my body and my organs:

Three days after I started to take one table spoon in the morning and in the evening, the body and the organs started to react. First, I believed negatively. As it is my nature, I remained firm with myself and continued to take „Superbiomin". The turning point came after five or six days. The **digestion, well-being, apetite, efficiency, physical** and **psychological state** improved every day. It is incredible, now, after seven weeks, I could work again for twenty hours without my élan going off.

During the period I have been taking „Superbiomin" my wife, my brothers and sisters, children and clients became aware of my energy and my élan and especially of my stamina and wanted an explanation for my physical state. All of them then wanted immediately to get some of this „Superbiomin".

One can hardly describe in writing what has happened inthe meantime. From **sleeplessness, arthritis, constipation, heartburn, indisposition, tiredness** to the unbelievable, in such a short period! Telephone calls and personal evidences came nearly every day.

It nearly blows up one's mind!

To make sure that you, too, learn about these experiences, it goes for me without saying, to inform you. My certificate for your product:

This natural product is a miracle of nature!

Mr. Dr. Werner M. from U./FRG writes:

Since the end of May, I have been taking your stone flour twice a day and I am very satisfied with the result. My **kidney stones** started to move and I hope to entirely get rid of these nuissance soon. You will receive information about the progress of my cure. I expect it will take three months.

Ms. Margarete St. from W./Austria writes:

In October 1977 I had a **collarbone fracture** after a car accident and was operated. For five years I got physical therapy, but my **shoulder** was always tensed-up and it hurt constantly – especially when the weather changes. I have now been taking your stone powder twice per day for about five weeks. The tensions and the **swelling** have disappeared and the shoulder does not hurt any more.

Ms. Anneliese F. from F./FRG writes:

I have been taking your stone flour since 1 May 1986. The **arthrosis** of my left knee has disappeared completely. I feel as if I was many years younger. I do hope it helps also many other people, just as it has helped me.

Ms. Mag. Johanna P. from W./Austria writes:

A month ago your „Superbiomin" was recommended to me – I have been taking it since that time regularly, and a few days ago I noticed a great recuperation of my hand. I now can fully stretch my thumb. (X-ray findings dated 11 March 1986 state: **arthropathy – „Herberden'sche Knoten"**).

Ms. P. K. from L./Austria writes:

I am now 51 years old, had a severe **loss of hair** and a **nervous disease**. Everything has gone. Now I feel as if I was 20 again.

Mr. Leopold St. from W./Austria writes:

I take the liberty to tell you the following about the use of the stone flour: A neighbour who, for a long time, could move only with the help of crutches, all of a sudden walked with just one stick. When I asked her which treatment she has had, she told me that a niece had provided her with the stone flour of which she has been taking, for several months, one teaspoon full in the morning and in the evening, and, therefore, is able now to move nearly without pain.

For several years I had not been able to lift my arms, could not comb myself, nor shave or wash my hair, it even happened at breakfast that I dropped my coffee cup. I went through all the varios treatments in different hospitals, but it did not bring any success worth mentioning. Since September 1986 I have been taking every morning one heaped teaspoon of this flour. Now, I can tell you honestly about my success. I am not only able again to move my arms easily, but also my entire **general health** has improved. I am able to read without spectacles also texts in small print. My wife even pointed out to me that I have again some **hair** on my bald head. I can drive a car or a bicycle without any difficulties.

Now that I have started to use the third kilogramme of your stone flour, I have to write this letter to you, and I can only highly recommend it to all those people who – like me – had already given up every hope.

Ms. Therese L. from A./FRG writes:

Today I am very anixous to write to you. First of all I would like to thank you very much for your efforts. Since May of this year I have been taking your stone flour which meanwhile has become so well-known. I can only stress that it does me very well. The great **giddiness** which I had suffered from for two years has disappeared, let alone the many sleepless nights that are now belonging to the past. My **general health** has improved tremendously. I feel better all together and, at present, do not need any medicines.

Mr. Dr. Heino G. from A./FRG writes:

You may be interested to learn that a friend of mine, professional, nearly 80 years old, has had the feeling, since Christmas, he was going to die. He was also in a pitiable state. After taking the stone flour, a change took place immediately: the agonizing **tiredness** disappeared. Moreover, a **kidney stone** that had troubled him for a long time started to move.

Ms. Gisela K. from G./Austria writes:

A short time ago (about three weeks), I received your „Superbiomin" and have obtained very good results. For example, my constant **colics** and my constant **ravenous hunger** have disappeared completely. So, one can lose weight much more easily. I am completely enthusiastic about this wonder drug.

Ms. Silvia E. from B./FRG writes:

My parents received your stone flour about ten weeks ago. They were so enthusiastic about it that they persuaded me to take it too. So I did. For years I have had difficulties with my **digestion** and I had to take a lot of medicines. But since I started to take your stone flour, I do not need them any more. I am very happy about this. Moreover, I feel much better.

Ms. Elly V. from B./Austria writes:

I received your parcel with thanks and have been taking, now for the third week, 3 x per day one teaspoon of the stone flour. The **colics** and the **itching** (head and body) and the **iron level** (here lies the cause for **giddi-**

ness, headache, tiredness, etc.) have improved considerably and I have no more **blurred fingers** and **tear sacks**, although I have been taking the stone flour just the third week. The **chronic diarrhoea** my husband used to suffer from, has completely disappeared.

Ms. C. Kluth from N./FRG writes:

Since taking „Superbiomin" (stone flour), he started to take it two months ago, my husband can move his **shoulders** just like in the times, when he was young. He is able again to do exercises on the horizontal bar and to swim excellently, i.e. he crawls.

Many thanks.

Ms. Albina H. from Sch./Austria writes:

Thank you very much for your prompt service. We all are just old and feeble wee wifeys. But it helps all of us. I myself am very satisfied. I just would like to inform you, an acquaintance has been suffering for years from **fistulas on the anus**. Suddenly they disappeared. We all are very happy.

Ms. Paula T. from I./Austria writes:

Every day I took a level teaspoon of the stone flour with some water. I have been suffering for some time from **lack of iron**, and therefore from **brittle finger nails**. I am an enemy of taking medicines, but the Biomin-stone flour has helped me.

Ms. F. and Mr. K. H. from B./FRG write:

We have been taking the stone flour every day and my doctor has already noted an improvement of my **metabolism**, since I still suffer from the poisens of my **typhoid fever**.

Ms. Waltraud L. from H./FRG writes:

Since I have a large circle of acquaintances – because of my profession of a head physician in the hospital – and they heard from me that I give to my husband who is three times a week under treatment with a special kidney machine (dialyzer), 2 x 1 teaspoon of this flour, these people too, want to try it out.

I myself have been taking it for the past three months and I feel extremely well.

My husband also takes it well and I am conviced that by the end of the year we can say, there is a good result. I keep all the chemical loboratory findings, in order to be able to deliver a correct proof, which values he had before starting to and when taking the stone flour. We have a firm belief in God. He has shown us this way, we will continue.

Ms. Ruth V. from St./FRG writes:

I received your stone flour at the beginning of July. I have to tell you that I had such a success which I hardly can describe. By now I have been taking the stone flour for exactly eight weeks and I must admit that I nearly feel healthy again.

My **arthrosis** in the knees has disappeared. For five years I could not descend the steps. Today I jump down the steps just like I did, when I was 20. My **periostitis** has disappeared completely, previously I had to take strong pain-killers every day for 3 years. Apart from that, my whole physical condition is excellent, I hardly can conceive it. Because of my **diabetes** I had such terrible pain in my legs and in hy hands – they have gone.

My acquaintance, who took the stone flour together with me, no longer suffers from **sciatic pains, disturbed circulation** in the legs, **headache** nor **nosebleed**, complaints that had troubled him for many years. He feels as if he was 20 years younger.

Mr. Dipl.-Ing. Johannes C. from K./FRG writes:

Your stone flour worked wonders. Five weeks after I started to take it, I suddenly could move again my arms and legs just like in the earlier days. I had walked with a stick and I had been unable to climb the stairs. Diagnosis: **Polyarthritis (rheumatism)**.

I, too, eat your „primary rocks powder". I already took 1 kg and I am very satisfied. I still have nearly another 2 kg, later on I will probably be able to remove mountains, because already now I feel extremely strong and well.

Ms. Johanna B. from N./FRG writes:

Since April 1980 I have been taking your stone flour, which you had sent to me and I can say I have had a great therapeutic success.

1. I used to have a lot of pain on both **soles of the foot**. After 14 days the pain had disappeared completely.

2. On all ten **finger-nails** I had a lot of white spots – a sign of **lack of iron**. This has gone back to normal by now, the spots have disappeared.

3. Four months ago I had terrible pain in both **shoulders** and I hardly could lift my hands to comb myself or to bind my apron on the back. No

medicine or ointment helped to alleviate this suffering. Taking this stone flour I got rid of these three terrible sufferings.

My sister, Ms. Resi A. from W./Austria had a lot of trouble with her **heart disease.** She had to swallow every day 3–4 heart tablets. Since taking the stone flour she no longer needs tablets. She is 73 and really comes to life again and feels well.

Mr. Erwin G. from D./Austria writes:

As to myself I can inform you that, after having taken 1 teaspoon of „Superbiomin" per day for three weeks, I got rid of the very inconvenient **itching of the skin**. This itching of the skin I feel immediately on my body, whenever the temperature of my body changes. It is a **metabolic disturbance**.

Ms. Margarete St. from W./Austria writes:

My **cholesterol concentration** before and after taking „Superbiomin":

	Overall cholesterol concentration	triglycerides	gamma G. t.	alkal. phosphates
1986–03–17:	312	213	86	314

On 1986–05–26 I started to take „Superbiomin":

1986–07–01:	298	180	61	300
1986–08–04:	257	129	44	218

This was checked by the family doctor, Dr. G. from W./Austria.

Ms. Elfriede Sch. from D./FRG writes:

I am 66 years old and had **depressions** for three years. After I had taken „Superbiomin" = stone powder, for eleven days, my depressions disappeared. My **loss of hair** stopped, my **backache** disappeared several weeks ago. I could not lift my arms any more. Now, everything is OK again. Today I am again full of the joy of living, thanks to your miracle-rock.

Ms. Else N. from D./FRG writes:

I took 2 teaspoons of your rock flow per day and I can only confirm that my complaints – **pain in the joints and in the back, bladder complaints** and **flutter** – got much better and partly have disappeared. I was born in 1918 and I am so glad that I can move again without pain and canwork energetically in the garden. My sincere thanks.

Ms. K. H. from W./Austria writes:

Since October 1985 I have been suffering from **pain in the back and from pain in the hip joints**, and I could not walk without a stick and without outside help. I got many injections and underwater massages, without much result. But, nevertheless, I have to be operated at the beginning of September, because I was burnt in spring 1968 by cobalt irradiation and my left **hip joint** was damaged and the head is missing.

Since 4 May 1986, I have been taking your „Superbiomin" every day in the morning and in the evening 1 teaspoon with some water – I was successful.

On 5 June I went to my hairdresser (I was picked up by a car and brought back). I had a permanent wave made. The hairdresser said she needed today much more curlers, your hair has grown and has turned darker (was already white). So I told her about the stone flour!

Then, from the middle of June, I could turn around a bit, lift the feet and put on my shoes by myself. The great pain has gone, now I only have slight pain, quite bearable.

Since I will get a new hip joint on my left foot, I can only tell you that I am happy that these severe pains have decreased!

I have several witnesses who know how badly I walked during the period from 23 December 1985 to 6 January 1986. My friend had totake me in tow, although I was walking with a stick.

Many thanks.

Ms. Juliane T. from W./Austria writes:

From an acquaintance I received a „taste", because the past 1 3/4 years I had to overcome a severe illness. Up to now I needed one Cortison injection every two weeks. Now, I have been feeling remarkably better, already for four weeks.

Ms. Gertrude W. from W./Austria writes:

For 16 years I have been suffering from **colics**, there was no remedy for it. Only those who experienced this themselves know how weak one feels. I did not believe one word of the reports I heard about your mineral flow, but I tried it thinking: „If it does not help, at least it won't harm." But then the big surprise came: it did help, namely 100%. No more pain, no more **colics**, I could forget the rigorous fasting days, which I had to insert from time to time.

Ms. Maria D. from B./Austria writes:

I am so happy! I have not been taking any medicine for three weeks, but taking 2 teaspoons of the mineral flow with $^{1}/_{4}$ water. For at least 20 years I have been suffering from **hypertension** and today I went to have my blood pressure measured, what a surprise for the doctor and for myself: instead of 180 I had only 110. It was like a miracle. Moreover, an acquaintance told me that they have been watering their gum tree with it and within 14 days it got seven new leaves. His wife got rid of her **rash**. I am glad that there are you and your mineral flow. Many hearty thanks!

Ms. Bertha L. from B./Austria writes:

Your valuable and for humanity so suitable „Superbiomin" has become also for me a „remedy" for the following reasons, which I want to tell you for your information.

I am happy to possess „Superbiomin" since 24 May 1986 and I take 2 teaspoons per day, because I want to reduce my **diabetic values** which I have had for 17 years and could not get rid of – despite all efforts with diets and physical movement. Years ago my diabetic values were so high that I was in coma with a diabetic value of 507 and was rescued by Prof. Dr. B. LKH L./Austria in the last moment. This was 1969. Since that time I have to balance this out with injections, but nevertheless, had from time to time values of 180 to 210.

Since taking „Superbiomin", my values dropped to 80 to 90, and have remained there, so that my doctor, Dr. L., whom I have been consulting regularly, was astonished about this success. Furthermore, my **blood pressure**, which used to vary constantly, went back to normal.

Moreover, I had for about four years, a **renal cyst** on the right side, that had been diagnosed by LKH L. and LKH G. by means of a flouroscopic examination which – according to the findings – could be removed only by an operation or by a puncture. I therefore had some pain and was sensitive to pressure. After I took „Superbiomin", this cyst has disappeared completely – no more swelling, let alone pain. I stress once again – according to findings – it was a big cyst.

Now that I am a healthy person, I am overjoyed, although I was „81 years" old on 29 April 1986.

Already a few days after I had started to take „Superbiomin", it began to work fully and heeled my complaints. This is proof enough – against the opinion of the pert persons – and the poor classical medicine has become a bit poorer, and with them the pharmacists and their like, who now may fear to lose customers. Before taking and after the examination of „Superbiomin", this only has amused my husband and myself considerably.

Furthermore we would like to wish you lots of luck and success and also such a good health.

Ms. Albina H. from Sch./Austria writes:

Once more I would like to ask you to send me „Superbiomin". I am very happy and content, that my **knees** are so good now and that I can sleep again during the night. I am also able again to lie on either side.

Mr. Lothar K. from L./FRG writes:

Your „Superbiomin" has helped my wife within a short time. She no longer has **hypertension** and the **noises in her ear** have also stopped. I myself also took the powder, and I feel relieved from a pressure.

Mr. Dir. Josef W. from F./Austria writes:

Since the beginning of July 1986 I have been taking the stone flour regularly and I volontarily make known the outcome.

The colour of my regrowing **hair** is noticeably darker. The **defaecation** has completely normalized. The **blood picture** (as established by my doctor three days ago) is excellent. The **general well-being** is remarkably good compared to the **tiredness** I had before.

But the greatest success of the stone flour: for years my **festering heels** (I am severely war-disabled and had an amputation on both heels) are clean and covered with a new skin, so the wounds are closed, although all medicines had failed all those years before. And even if the Ministry of Health has prohibited the sale of this unique stone flour as a medicine, its heeling success cannot be denied.

I continue to take it just like my acquaintances who had also very good results with the **blood picture**, got rid of **constipation**, and, in one case, reduction of the **gout** of the hands and relief of pain was achieved.

Ms. Maria K. from L./FRG writes:

I have been taking 2 teaspoons of „Superbiomin" for the past five weeks regularly and you may see that I am already better able to write with my very **gouty hands**. At the beginning the **digestion** was dark, nearly black, then – because of my severe **damage of the liver** – nearly white and for approximately the last ten days it turned normal again. My high **blood pressure** dropped already a bit. You really have helped me a lot.

Ms. Ursula W. from H./FRG writes:

My husband has taken the bio-band from the middle of June until September 1986, and has had good success. His **arm** that has been hurting for years, expecially when he made certain movements, has improved considerably. I myself could take „Superbiomin" only for eight weeks, but I too have had good results, especially with the **defaecation**.

Mr. George N. from M./FRG writes:

I regard the stone flour as a kind of earth and as a gift of God, because it has helped me considerably and I want to confirm this herewith.

Since 1961 already I have been suffering from **hypertension** and **cardiac insufficiency**, both diseases constantly grew worse.

In 1978 I even went to a nonmedical practitioner for treatment at the same time as I went to my family doctor.

In 1979 I could be kept alive in hospital only with the help of a cardiac pacemaker.

In 1980 I had water in the lungs and I could only be kept alive with oxygen, the same happened again in the year 1981.

In 1982 I had a **prostate** operation and the **diabetic values** were also elevated.

In 1983 I got **rheumatism** in my right arm and inthe year 1984 I could hardly move it at all and I could hardly drive my car.

Now I have been taking your stone flour since May 1986 and I nearly have no more complaints, everything is normal and at the age of 75 I feel as if I was 57. Your esteemed daughter can confirm this, she saw me, when I came to your firm. I will continue to treat myself with it.

Mr. Johannes G. from F./FRG writes:

I am 46 years old and have been suffering since 1975 most of the time from **depressions**, that can turn very bad. Maybe you will know that depressive patients tend, in the most severe cases, permanently to attempted suicides.

About two months ago I bought from you 26 kg „Superbiomin". Whenever I take a teaspoon of this powder, my **depressions** are gone for several days completely. I hardly can believe this myself, since I have had plenty of experience with the respective medicines (psychopharmacologic drugs).

I am grateful to you with all of my heart.

Ms. Ingeborg Sch. from Ü./FRG writes:

I would like to let you know how well I am, now, after having taken „Superbiomin" for three months. Today I received from my doctor the information, that I have a blood like a young lady. My **leucocytes** have also increased. I am, after all, 72 years old. This really is a fine thing. But I cannot understand, why this wonderful remedy has been prohibited in our country. This is probably due to the pharmacy.

Even my horses like it very much, one can notice it in them.

I will continue to put it into the food of my horses and will distribute it also among my friends.

A friend of mine had your stone flour analyzed by two nonmedical practitioners and had it also measured with a pendulum. It finds recognition everywhere. We all are very grateful to you.

Ms. Ursula Dorothee L. from B./FRG writes:

I can hardly put it into words to let you know, how well I feel after having taken „Superbiomin". Although I am already 66 years old, I have been working now for eight months in my old profession as a secretary in a notary's office, and I am working every day up to 12 hours, without any difficulties. I attribute these reserves of strength entirely to your remedy. This improvement is especially remarkable, since I was quite dead-beat, even exhausted and had a lot of pain. This belongs to the past, since I started to take „Superbiomin" regularly.

Press Articles

„Neue Welt" reports:

The Wonder-Earth from Austria.
Facts behind the Super-Powder!

Robert Schindele (54), who by now is known all over the world, is sure of his matter. He believes that his miracle powder of rock flow brings the „everlasting youth", but at least turns the biological time for 20 to 30 years back. BILD wrote about this in headlines, television reported it. But what is really behind this magma rock that the smart veneer wood manufacturer from Gansback-Kicking in Lower Austria now sells in tons as stone flour all over the world? Well, meanwhile the miracle powder „Superbiomin" is sought after not only in Austria and in Germany. Even King Fahd from Saudi Arabia wants to have Schindele's miracle-earth. The price does not matter. There are orders from China, Australia, Israel and from the USA.

NEUE WELT got the chemical analysis of this magma rock. Indee: it contains 22 minerals, many of them are even vital. The six most important are silicic acid, potassium, calcium, iron, magnesium and zinc. **Germany's most famous nonmedical practitioner, Dr. Manfred Köhlechner,** has been recommending it for several years already, to those, who wish to feel younger, more energetic and healthier. This is produced by the following six minerals:

○ **Silicic acid:** It is described by naturopathy as a primary substance of life. It supports the **respiration** of our **cells** and makes sure that the **cells** do not age so quickly. It influences the **skin, hair, nails** and **muscles**. Moreover it stimulates the **digestion**.

○ **Potassium:** It is important for the **supply of blood of the cardiac muscle** and of other **muscles**. Finally it regulates the **blood pressure** and dehydrates. So, it keeps our **heart** going and makes the body slim.

○ **Calcium:** This element is very important for the health of our **bones** and our **teeth**. Calcium also strengthens our **connective tissue**, which is responsible for the **youthfulness** of the body. If calcium is missing, then especially women often feel lifeless, tired and nervous. As of the age of 40, calcium is anyway important for every woman.

○ **Iron:** It is responsible for a sufficient supply of oxygen in the **blood**. Lack of iron makes women look pale and feel exhausted.

○ **Magnesium:** This mineral is of utmost importance to our **heart**. It protects us from **overstrain** and **stress**. 400 milligrammes per day are sufficient.

○ **Zinc:** It gets the **metabolism** going and strengthens the **cells**. If zinc is missing the **hair** fall out, wounds heal badly, women cannot have babies any more.

Another Press Report:

University Clinic Considers „Superbiomin" to be a Universal Remedy!

KICKING. – Although the sale of „Superbiomin" as a medicine is still prohibited in Austria and in FRG the reports of success about the good results achieved with the primary rock flow do not stop.

At the first international fair for a more human environment, which took place in Strasbourg (France) in August, Schindele received for his primary rock flow the „Medaille d'Or" (gold medal).

The number of medals that were awarded alltogether were only ten . . .

It does not indicate, whether this gold medal was awarded for the primary rock flow as a medicine for human beings or as a fertilizer for the soil and trees respectively.

A great „songs of praise" for „Superbiomin" also comes from Switzerland, from the national Cooperating University of America N. C. in Cham (Switzerland).

This university clinic employs, with great success, in addition to their system and method (athermic pulsing electronic magnetic high frequency fields and waves generator) the „high grade bio-minerals from the Haus Schindele".

Especially for reduced formation of callus after **fracture** (time reduced by 60%), against all **rheumatic diseases** and – this may astonish – against **cardiac infarct** „Superbiomin" is „the" remedy! Now it is being tested as to its effect on **nervous diseases**.

Maria Bruckner

„Canada Kurier 1986" reports:

Stone Flour „Superbiomin" now Available also in Canada!

WINNIPEG. – The „miraculous earth" from Austria, which is obtained from a wacke rich of mineral elements, and which has already created a great stir in Europe as a natural remedy, is now available also in Canada. It is sold under the trade name „Superbiomin" by the firm Super Biomin Canada Inc., in Winnipeg, which has obtained the selling rights for North America. The first retailer to sell this stone flour ist the German-Canadian shop Neumann's Fine Jewellery Ltd. in Winnipeg, Man. and Kelowna B. C.

Everything started in the beautiful Wachau, Lower Austria, in Kicking, a village of about 50 soals. The veneer wood manufacturer and forest owner Robert Schindele, 54, discovered three years ago the surprising effects of a rock deposit in his forest. Suddenly trees that were dying, were green again and shot forth. The reason: During construction works they had gotten into touch with the dust of the stones.

Schindele had the stones analyzed, after that he swallowed the powder in the morning and in the evening. He experienced himself, according to the reports, the beneficial effects of the „miracle drug". Gout and colics disappeared, his sparce and white hair turned dark again and thick. His **blood pressure** too improved and dropped from 180 to 145, not to mention the diminished **virility**.

Robert Schindele refuses to call it a „wonder drug", as it was denoted in many European journals. He maintains that his rock flow simply contains the absolutely right mixture of minerals of which are 22 mineral elements, among others the six most important ones, that make you feel more healthy, more vital and younger: silicic acid, potassium, calcium, iron and zinc.

„Since the fields, on which the food is grown, the soils, eluviate, and are fed up only by artificial substances, human beings virtually have to fall ill" Mr. Schindele declares. Or, on the other hand, they can get healthy again, if they make use of the gift of the nature from the quarry. By the way it is a special magma rock, that does not exist anywhere else in the world, so they say.

In a German magazin the medical doctor from Munich, Dr. Peter Schleicher, remarked about the rock flow with the name „Superbiomin": „It certainly helps a lot of people, because silicic acid, for example, detoxicates the liver and purifies the blood. It eliminates the consecutive symptoms of vaccinations and takes effect against head ache. It strengthens generally the **nails** and the **connective tissue**. Aluminium oxide helps against **indigestions**. Anyway, it contains important means for the body like zinc, magnesium and molybdenum. There is often a lack in the body, if it is attakked by severe illnesses like **cancer**. Phosphorus supports the circulation of the blood. Potassium, natrium and magnesium are of great importance for the cells."

„Blick ins Land" reports:

Superbiomin: From a Healthy Soil, Over Healthy Plants and Animals to Healthy Human Beings!

One day they discovered in the woodlands of the veneer wood manufacturer Schindele an alleged roadstone, which behaved in a very peculiar way. When it was raining, it started to gradually dissolve, until it disappeared completely – and with it the entire surface. They had this strange wacke that crumbled in the hand analyzed by scientists and they came to surprising results.

Tests and analyses proved that this material contains all vital minerals and trace elements and, moreover, is free from toxic substances. When ground to powder, it proves to be by far superior to other stone flours, because of this composition, but also, mainly, because of its high content of potassium and its ability to quilt.

The practical proof:
When the road was built, a fine dust was produced which covered the surrounding trees with a thin layer, and one could observe – certainly also due to the dissolved rock which acted as a fertilizer – an enormous recovery of the trees that grew along the street. Especially with fir trees that show today six completely healthy generations of needles.

The Vital Trace Elements

The natural food contains trace elements in varying concentration and of different physical and chemical forms. Today an element is considered useful for the organism and for the preservation of health, if a measurable lack of this element in the food reduces the growth or the fitness of the human being, animal or plant in a „reproducible manner". So, also toxic elements like arsenic, cadmium, lead and probably also aluminium are, in very small quantities, necessary for the cell metabolism, although they can be toxic in higher concentrations.

Trace Elements

Element	mg/kg
Natrium	195.0
Copper	37.2
Zinc	85.9
Cobalt	18.3
Molybdenum	0.1
Boron	9.8
Chromium	85.8
Nickel	40.6
Vanadium	69.5

Mineral Content

30%	Alkali feldspar
20–30%	Plagioclase
20–30%	Quartz
15–20%	Biotite
5–10%	Disthene, Garnet, Silimanite

Accessory Materials:
Ore, Zircon, Rutile

Extract from an expertise: „This rock deposit is a para-gneiss in a special state of maintenance, which is found only in ledges with the same primary rock and similar strain. Important for the effect of the rock flow is, apart from the minerals is contains, the special solution behaviour of the minerals and the transformation, respectively, into other mineral elements, whereby certain atoms and molecules are released. This rock flow is characterized by its rapid effect and its long repository effect."

This probably unique rock is ground to powder in a mammoth mill of the mineral factory Schindele, and sold as a fertilizer under the trade-name SUPERBIOMIN Flora.

It is applied with great success for fertilizing forests, for fertilizing the soil, as an addition to manure, as well as for the professional and hobby horticulture. SUBERPIBOMIN also has an excellent effect on indoor plants.

„Bildwoche" reports an 26 April 1986:

Since we have been Taking this Powder, we Feel Many Years Younger!

By Wolf-Rüdiger Goertz and Thomas Ruddies (photographs)

Forest officers write from USA and even Australia. Germans come in their car and take with them a 40 kg-bag. They have different reasons, but they all want exactly the same thing from Robert Schindele, 54, from Kicking in the Wachau: stone flour. He tried it himself. First against the dying of the woods, later (by chance) also against his diseases. Followers swear: „Since we have been taking this powder, we feel many years younger."

The story of the heeling powder started in July 1981. Veneer wood manufacturer Schindele: „At that time we were constructing a path through the woodland." They mecadamized the path with lumps of stone from the side slopes. The dust penetrated the surrounding. After a few weeks the surprising result: dying coniferous woods shot forth again!

Vienna discovered the secret: The powder contains an extremely high share of minerals: 18.3% aluminium oxide, 7.8% potassium oxide, 1.4% magnesium oxide as well as the trace elements natrium, manganese, cobalt, nickel. There are no traces at all of the toxic led or cadmium. Soil and trees recover because of this „fertilizer".

But the sensation about this heeling magma rock was created 1985, when Prof. Graefe of the Academy of Science in Vienna told Mr. Schindele, who was seeking his advice, more or less for fun:

„These minerals could also help you." From that moment Schindele swallowed every day two teaspoons of the rock flow: „My **attacks of**

gout disappeared rather quickly. The **uric acid level** dropped from 7.5 to 2.3. My **colesterol** disappeared.” The family doctor Dr. Tavakollan will talk in May on television about the medical history and cure of Mr. Schindele. Furthermore, ten people have been testing the stone flour for half a year under medical supervision.

Many acquaintances of Mr. Schindele, who took the powder, do not need this any more. Erich Mittendorfer from Melk: the **attacks of gout** I used to suffer from in my toes, have disappeared completely.” Edeltraud Bauer from Mauer bei Loosburg: My **bones** used to hurt. The pain has stopped.”

Dr. Walter Herbel, chief of the „Chemisches Untersuchungsamt” of the University of Hamburg believes it to be necessary, to have the powder analyzed scientifically, but he also thinks that its effect is comparable to the effect of mineral element preparations.

„Bild der Frau” reports an 21 April 1986:

Köhnlechner: This is How the Miraculous Earth Really Rejuvenates!

Does the Austrian miracle earth, the newspapers have been reporting about it for several days, really rejuvenate and make healthier? I am asked repetedly. I know people who advanced their leave over night, just to go to the Waldviertel in Lower Austria and to buy in a stock of the miracle earth from the wood manufacturer and factory owner Schindele. Does it really pay?

I got a chemical analysis of this earth. It really contains 22 minerals, many of which are vital.

The six most important mineral elements are „old acquaintances”, which I have been recommending for 14 years to all those who want to become younger, healthier and more vital: silicic acid, potassium, calcium, iron, magnesium, zinc.

I can only confirm:

This earth can cause miracles, especially for women. I will soon explain why. The most important: Get immediately into your car and get, like many others, a bag full of this earth from Austria. These minerals that cause the miracle in the miracle earth you can also get in nearly every pharmacy – individually or composed, according to your wishes. This is how the six minerals act:

○ **Silicic acid:** In naturopathy it is called „primary substance of life”. It furthers the respiration of the cells and takes care that the cells do not age so quickly. Visible signs: skin, hair and nails stay youthful. The muscles remain elastic for a longer time. Moreover, silicic acid stimulates the digestion. Diarrhoea or constipation disappear. If applied externally (as a gel), it heels wounds, pimples, muscular pains and pains in the joints.

○ **Potassium:** It effects a better supply of blood of the cardiac muscle, regulates the blood pressure, stimulates dehydration. It keeps the heart young and the body slim.

○ **Calcium:** It is very important for healthy, strong bones and teeth. They do not age so quickly and do not get brittle and fragile prematurely. Moreover calcium strengthens the connective tissue, which is vital for the body to stay young. Lack of calcium causes, especially with women, sleeplessness, nervousness. As of the age of 40 calcium is decisive for every woman, whether she ages faster or stays young for a longer time.

○ **Iron:** It makes sure that sufficient oxygenic blood is available. Lack of iron makes women pale, feeble, tired, susceptible to infections. Women lose a lot of iron during their monthly period.

○ **Magnesium:** gallop rhythm, circulatory disturbances, cramps in the calf of the leg in the night, blood clots that cause thrombosis – all this is caused by the lack of magnesium. This mineral is absolutely basic, it ensures that our heart remains young and that the arteries do not become brittle that blood clots do not cause a sudden cardiac infarct. Especially women who are on slimming diet, often suffer from lack of magnesium. They get slim, but they age twice as fast. All those who slim or eat a lot of protein, need to add magensium to their diet, in order remain young and fit.

○ **Zinc:** It gets the metabolism of the body going, fortifies the cells. If zinc is missing, the hair fall out, women often can no longer have babies any more, woonds heel badly, the body is more susceptible to diseases. Attention: Every time she is subject to psychological stress, a woman loses particularly much zinc.

You can see, how important these minerals of the Austrian miracle earth are. Make sure you get enough of it and you will really remain longer young, longer healthy.

„Bild der Frau" reports on 28 April 1986:

This is How you Can Obtain the Miracle Earth

It Makes Skin and Hair Beautiful and Helps Against Monthly Pain (Algomenorrhea)!

By Sigi Kopp

No wonder. Everybody wants now to have this miracle earth that is said to rejuvenate. For a week the telephone of the wood manufacturer Schindele who discovered, under his forest, the rock containing a lot of minerals, is constantly occupied by day and by night. Hundreds of people phone BILD der FRAU: How can we get this miracle earth? The addresses are listed at the bottom of this page. First of all some news.

The pharmacist Dr. Ernst Dieter Prinzenberg from Bochum has analyzed the ground rock flow from Schindele's woods, and confirmed its heeling effect especially on women.

„My miracle earth makes the skin more beautiful", Mr. Schindele says. Dr. Prinzenberg: „This comes from the high content of silicic acid in combination with zinc. They strengthen the hair cells, can effect new growth. It is possible that hair that turned grey too early regains its natural colour."

„My miracle earth helps against monthly pain", Mr. Schindele says. Dr. Prinzenberg: „Untimely, too long or missing monthly periods can be influenced positively by these minerals."

You can find out in which phamacies and in which health food shop of your region you can buy already next week the miracle earth (250 g ca. DM 10) from the representations listed below.

„Bildzeitung" reported in April 1986:

Miracle Stone: 70-Year-Old: „Tie me Down, I am so Strong!" Also the Chinese want the Miracle Stone!

By Christian Sturm

„Tie me Down!" the engineer Johannes Drachsler shouted. „Tie me Down – I am so strong. I do not know what to do with my strength!" Mr. Drachsler is 70 years old. He took the powder, that is won from the „miracle stone". It is said to make people „20 to 30 years younger" (BILD reported). Many people order the stone powder by the hundredweight.

Mr. Drachsler, who has a car workshop in Schall-Emmersdorf told BILD: Previously I always felt tired and lifeless, I had pain in the lung." Two months ago he started to take regularly the brown stone powder – one teaspoon with water in the morning and one teaspoon in the evening. Drachsler: „Now I go to my workshop already at six o'clock in the morning – before I went at eight o'clock. Now I work in the evening until 8 pm – after that I go to the pub."

At one of the evenings in the pub Mr. Drachsler full of the joy of living shouted to his friends: „Tie me down!" Now he has discovered another way to live his youthful buoyance to the full: „I walk again in the mountains. I feel strong and lively."

Ms. Lydia Sch. (76), pensioner, had a similar experience. „I cook, wash, clean and iron for a family of five. In the evening I used to go to bed at 9 dead tired. Now I stay up until 11 o'clock and watch TV without falling asleap."

The news of the alleged rejuvenating effect of the miracle stone went around the world.

The wood manufactuerer Robert Schindele (54), who is the owner of the query with the wonder rock, already had enquiries from India and China. One banker from the USA ordered two metric hundredweights, a German from Bocholt who was on holiday in Portugal, phoned from his hotel: „I would like to have 10 kg!"

A veterinarian from Varel ordered by telephone 120 to 160 pounds: „I am 56 years old and certainly suffer from symptoms of old age. But first I want to try out the stone powder on my animals." This, the farmer Gustav H. (45) from St. Leonhard has already done: „I gave it to my peacocks, now they have a very specially shining plumage."

„Kurier" reported on 23 June 1986:

Disputed Stone Flour for Germans „Healthy"!

MELK/KICKING. – While the native medical doctors still carry out private warfares on professional criticism about the utility or valuelessness of the stone flour „Superbiomin", the producer of the „wonder drug", Robert Schindele, called the expert opinion of a German expert from the official food control agency. They very officially confirmed not only that his mineral cure is not only a „real food" and is free from toxic, harmful substances, but, moreover, also that the mineral elements it contains build the basis for the functioning of the cells and the tissue.

The **formation of blood** is stimulated and the minerals are involved to a high degree, in the functioning and the formation of hormons, vitamins and enzymes. They are, in the first place, the main components for the **bones, teeth** and of special tissues of utmost importance which the body absolutely needs, otherwise this causes deficiency diseases.

Thus as stated in the expertise.

„But how about the **radioactivity** of the stone flour?" The producer had this anxious question of many customers also checked, and Schindele would not be Schindele, if he would not make capital even out ofthis fear from radioactivity: He put the examination results on the table, the iodine-

131 and the caesium-137 values are below the limit of detection. He even took the „offensive" in this direction:

„The boron (B) in the rock flow (0.006 milligrammes per gramme) has, on the contrary, an effect that prevents **antinotoxemia** or reduces it." Thus his statement, which he supported by a spectucular project in aid: He donated one ton of his rock flow for the victims of the reactor catastrophe in Tchernobyl. Already within the next few days – according to Schindele – the shipment will leave for USSR.

Johann Frank

„Bildwoche" reports on 24 April 1986:

Two kilogrammes reserved for everybody.
Excursion to the Miraculous powder!

Next week the first bus from Elite-Reisen will leave Hamburg for the first miraculous powder cure tour to the Wachau, Austria. This one week tour costs DM 588.– and includes two kilogrammes of the powder from the heeling magma rock from the heart of the earth.

The miraculous powder has been reserved specially for the cure tourists, because Robert Schindele, 54, who possesses the exclusive rights for exploitation, has temporarily stopped the production: „We are having examined at the moment, if the radioactive rain, that fell on the quarry has contaminated the magma rocks."

The Austrian is precautious, especially because some firms in Germany offer the so-called miracle powder, without possessing the selling rights. Schindele indignant: „I do not know which powder they sell at excessive prices."

In the meantime the first medical intermediary result is available. The head physician Dr. Abdul Aburumieh, examined his **blood** after his two-week powder cure: „My **cholesterol level** has not decreased." He now wants to wait for the results of his patients to whom he had recommended this miracle powder. The head physician: „I am by no means disappointed that it did not work at the first attempt." The members of his family continue to take the powder.

These days, ten persons are going to receive a letter from the Austrian television, informing them that they were selected to participate in a one-year miracle powder test under medical surveillance. Ten out of thousends who had applied. The letters filled half of a 20 square meters large office...

Helene Mühlwisch

„Die Welt" reports on 8 April 1986:

After the „Rock Flow Cure" Thirty Years Younger!

Kurt Pollak, Vienna

In Austria one seems to have come a huge step closer tothe age-old wish to attain eternal youth. As it happens often with decisive discoveries for the welfare of mankind, it was also this time that coincidence played the essential part, when the forest owner and veneer wood manufacturer Robert Schindele (54) from the village Kicking-Gansbach in the Wachau (Lower Austria), discovered the „rejuvenating tonic".

Robert Schindele seems to have found the „philosophers' stone", when, four years ago, he had a forest road covered with crushed rock, to be able to use his wood vehicles also under bad weather conditions. At the beginning of October 1985 he realized, much to his own astonishment, that fir trees, spruce trees and deciduous trees standing along the forest road and that were very much impaired, miraculously recovered completely. The forest owner informed the appropriate forest authority, who ordered a geological examination of the rocks. They come from a quarry that also belongs to Robert Schindele.

They found out that the stones contained a high portion of potassium and manganese. The scree material, containing minerals was obviously responsible for the regeneration of the dying trees. Wind and rain had contributed their share, that the rock flow got from the crushed-stone road into the woods, where it took effect as a „wonder-fertilizer". Today the forest region at the Jauerling, north of the Danube, can be considered as having been saved.

But two days ago the Austrian came up with a new sensation. His stone flour containing minerals, could not only save forests, this he believed to be able to prove, but it could also turn back the biological clock of the human being for 20 to 30 years. He experienced it himself, and again this happened just by chance: The man who had been troubled for several years by **gout** and had snow-white hair heard from a friend, a medical doctor, that he took every day one point of a knife of the rock flow, to keep his vitality. Thereupon Schindele made himself a „guinea pig" and swallowed his stone flow which was a good forest fertilizer, in larger dosages.

After a three-month „rock flow-cure" Robert Schindele reported yesterday about the outcome to WELT: „A real rejuvenation miracle came about me. Not only my **gout complaints** disappeared completely, but also the chronic **colics** I had been suffering from for twenty years, due to a **meat poisoning**, stopped.

The so wonderfully rejuvenated forest owner who does not want to get the reputation of a charlatan or a shrewd businessman, consulted some medical doctors who certified his astonishing rejuvenation and then reached themselves for the miracle drug. Since that time there was a deluge of letters of thanks from all over the world. And since it has been known that the mineral rock with a high content of molybdenum works wonders as a **remedy against disturbances of the potency**, Schindele was swamped with requests for his remedy.

Schindele who sells the miraculous rock at a ridiculously low price is, according to many „rejuvenated", absolutely due for the Nobel price. That the consumption of this „rejuvenating tonic" may cause detriments to the health or delayed consequences, Schindele denies, and refers to several medical doctors. In the meantime he has applied for a patent for his rock flow at the Austrian patent office.

„Praline" reports:

The „stone-wonder" from Gansbach-Kicking in Austria makes as fit as a fiddle (the customers) and rolling in (the quarry owner)!

„It is good for the sexual potency!" is the opinion of a Mercedes driver from Hamburg, and he bought in Austria 50 kg of the miraculous stone flour!

○ The quarry owner Schindele (54) tells personally to PRALINE how he got again good blood values and a good digestion.

○ PRALINE asked the people who queue up to buy and pay in cash, what hopes they have.

They „pilgrim" in masses, long lines of cars move patiently driving at a walking pace just like at a border to Italy during the holiday season. The destination of these „pilgrims" is Gansbach-Kicking, a tiny village not far from Melk in Lower Austria. They come from Brussels, Bremen, Zurich, Amsterdam to buy the miracle stone powder that is supposed to bring eternal youth.

Reports in German newspapers and magazins have caused a real stone-hysteria. Robert Schindele (54), the „inventor" of the polygenous that is ground to powder, does not know how this could happen all of a sudden.

PRALINE wanted to know how this wacke-boom could occur at all.

First of all a sitrep: Saturday 9 am. A lot of cars pile up in front of a huge storehouse, most of them are from the Federal Republic of Germany. In the warehouse a crowd. The waiting crowd is seized by a restlessness, because somebody spread the rumour that there was only a limited amount left.

Mrs. Schindele can hardly keep up with putting the heaps of hundred and thousandmark-bills into the drawer of her kitchen table, on which she makes out the bills. Most of them buy the stone flour in sacks of 40 kg.

An older woman from Hanover can hardly wait. She tears open the paper sack, takes a spoon full of the stone flour and puts it into a thermos flask. She fills a tumbler with the brownish liquid and drinks it absorbedly in small sips.

When asked what she expects from it she answers PRALINE: „There is nothing better for the stomach and the bowels. I know it from a friend of mine."

An elegantly dressed gentleman of about 50 years who dragged graspingly a sack to his Mercedes with a license number from Hamburg said, with a wink in his eye: „It's to be terrific for the **sexual potency**!"

Robert Schindele as a rule does not wish to speak to anybody, the telephone has been turned off for some time. But he has time for PRALINE.

We accompany him with some scientists to the quarry, which is the source of his new wealth. There we could be convinced that there is no reason to buy it for hoarding: Here are stored some estimated 20 million tons of first class primary rocks.

This is how the miraculous effect of the polygenous was first discovered: Robert Schindele had the forest roads in his wood covered with crushed stone. In doing so dust clouds developed and spread at a certain distance.

In this area something astonishing happened: The fir trees which had already been damaged by the acid rain so severely that they should be felled in the near future, recovered in the parts of the wood which had been covered by the stone dust, within a year, they again got new green needles.

Professor Dr. Johannes Mayer and Professor Dr. Graefe from the Austrian Academy of Science confirm to PRALINE: „There is no doubt that the recuperation of the trees is due to the stone flour."

As to the effect of his wacke on human beings Robert Schindele declares: „I used to suffer from gout, my hair was snow-white, the blood values poor. For several months I have been taking the stone powder, one teaspoon in the morning and in the evening, dissolved in water.

You can see for yourself: My hair gets slowly darker, also my **gout pains** have disappeared, as well as my colics, my skin has become smoother and my **blood values** are again super."

This was also confirmed by the head physician Dr. Aburumieh from

Melk: „It is correct what Mr. Schindele says. I now make myself experiments with the stone flour. In a few weeks I will be able to tell you more. The enormous amount and extraordinary content of minerals in the wacke makes me suppose that there is a very positive effect."

A German big businessman offered seven million DM to the Austrian for the general agency. But the father of four children declined the offer, he wants to trade his product himself.

No wonder, every day hundreds of orders are received, a. o. from about 600 medical doctors from all around the world.

Robert Schindele is confident: „I practically can supply the whole mankind with my product!"

Johann Frank reports:

Supplier of Stone Flour Does Not Yet Give Up

Expertise and Gold as New Triumphs

KICKING, MELK. – Robert Schindele is not allowed to sell his primary rocks flour either in Austria or in Germany as a medicine. But this prohibition has never forced the smart businessman from Kicking (district Melk) to his knees.

With three new triumphs he wants to prove his seriosity: At the fair „Human Environment – Futura 86" in Strasbourg (France) he received last August the international prize for his stone flour „Superbiomin", the gold medal. (Here also the trend-setting technique of a hydrogen operated car received the same distinction.)

The second ace he has „in his sleeve" is the confirmation he received from an American University Clinic in Switzerland. There „Superbiomin" was tested scientifically and really surprising therapeutic successes were achieved.

Finally Schindele sued through his lawyer against the prohibition to sell in Germany because of unconstitutionality. At the same time as he placed this formal objection, he requests by civil suit from the German government a damage of more than a million (DM).

The national „University of America N. C.", which has its seat in Cham (Switzerland), where a special technique of treatment, which was developed by NASA, is used successfully since 1973 (only patients are treated who did not respond to the various pharmacon programmes), add to their treatment with the system also „Superbiomin".

Their report astonishes: „After **fractures** the time for the heeling process is reduced by 60%; after a **cardiac infarct** there is a faster strengthening of the cardiac muskel, the **blood pressure** is also regulated rapidly. With acute and chronically inflamed processes of the soft-parts and with **joint diseases** a faster reduction of the pain is reached and an increase of the moveability of the **joints**.

The full professor of this university even recommends to every growing person to add from childhood minerals as a daily supplement to the food, to see a healthier generation grow up. Insurances and health insurances would see cost reduced to a great extent.

Five kilometers from Kicking a German couple from Frankfurt were guests in a village inn on the day of the KURIER-investigations. They expressly travelled 800 km to get the stone flour.

„Die Welt" reports:

Enormous Echo to the Mineral Cure!

Kurt Pollak, Vienna

Thousands of people from all parts of Germany are now on the search for youth and health. Among them are hundreds of readers of DIE WELT, who had learned in the issue of 8 April that the veneer wood manufacturer and forest owner Robert Schindele has discovered by chance a „rejuvenating tonic" in the form of a rock flow, containing minerals that might not only stop the worldwide dying of the woods, but also turn back the biological clock of the human beings for 20 to 30 years.

Robert Schindele believes to be able to prove that he could notice a really sensational **rejuvenation** of his body, after he started to swallow this rock flow that had already proved to be an excellent fertilizer for the forests. His hair that was up to then snow-white started to darken, his **gouty complaints** diminished suddenly, his up to then bad **blood values** are normal again.

Since the public found out about this „rejuvenating cure", the house of Robert Schindele, which is surrounded by woods and fields, and is situated in the village Gansback-Kicking, virtually became a Mecca for sick persons and patients, but also for speculators.

Astonishingly highly interested in this rock flow are medical doctors, pharmacists and representatives of pharmaceutical combines, the mineral composition of the rock flow is without parallel. A pharmaceutical firm in Washington has already ordered two shiploads of the polygenous.

The quarry in the Wachau is about 1 $^{1}/_{2}$ kilometers long and about 200 meters wide, it houses about 20 millions of tons of this polygenous. Schindele says: „I can supply practically the whole mankind with my rejuvenating tonic." And it looks as if he really will have to do so, since the world found out that the village Gansbach-Kicking is, in the first place, a „Fountain of Youth" also for people with little money in their wallet.

From the hundreds of letters that reach Robert Schindele every day, one can pick out human fates. Old, severely ill people, gather new hope.

An 87 year-old woman from Hamburg wrote: „I do feel absolutely healthy, but I just would like my white hair to turn black again, as it was, when I was young." A farmer from the area of Cologne wrote: „I survived three **cardiac infarcts** and suffer from bone atrophy. Please send me 100 kg of your rock flow." But also healthy people ask for it, because they suffer from **disturbances of potency**, or from sparce growth of hair.

Robert Schindele became over night involuntarily the „guru" of many people looking for hope. Together with his wife and his daughter he packs up the rock flow by day and by night and brings it to the post office. Since yesterday he also has to handle orders from the Austrian travel agencies, because hundreds of Germans who pass their holidays in Austria, turned to them and threaten they would never again come to Austria, if they did not get the „rejuvenating fluid".

A women's magazin from Hamburg approached Schindele with the request to make available some hundreds of kilogrammes for their readers, who hope, if they take „Superbiomin", they do not need a face lifting. Another German magazin wants to induce a notable, old actor to be a „guinea pig" for ten weeks, to become young again themselves.

Geologists and medical doctors who tried the rock flow themselves, unanimously said: „It seems that this polygenous is a discovery for the well-being of mankind, of flora and fauna."

„NÖN Bezirk Krems" 1986 reports:

Great Crush in Kicking: Stone Flour a Miraculous Drug?

KICKING (k.n.) – „Do you know, where the stone-flour-farmer lives?" I had stopped my car to ask, when I realized I could answer it myself. Some cart loads of wacke in front of the first house on the road Kochholz – Gansback and numerous cars, parking in front of the house revealed that this was the place I have been looking for.

Robert Schindele from Kicking whose name is now already well known in all of Central Europe, handles the sale of his stone flour at present in a rather improvised and primitive manner. This will change soon:

The stone flour has now received the name „Super-Biomin". „To be taken also against **chronic diseases**." On a yellowed piece of paper written by hand, that lies next to the cash register one can get more information: Against **problems with the growth of hair, metabolic disturbance, uric acid, circulatory insufficiency, colesterol, blood pressure troubles, weakness of the gums, bad digestion** etc. and so on. Schindele believes his completely white **hair** starts to turn blackish. The inhabitants of Kicking say, a bit sceptically and jealously, one should look a bit more carefully...

More than 20 different trace elements were identified in a chemical analysis and listed on the sack. Now the head physician from Melk, Dr. Aburumieh came „to the help" of Mr. Schindele with the declaration that he could prove the heeling effect on volontary test persons who had taken the stone flour. „This Biomin could, may be, even replace pharmaceutical medicines", he said to a „press-man".

A customer wanted to know from another customer, if it had helped him too. He has been taking now for several weeks twice a day one teaspoon. „I feel as strong as an ox" was the answer, „a small one!"

„Bildwoche" reports in May 1986:

Wrinkles Gone Through Wonder Powder

A searching glance in the mirror... and a content smile. Margarete Aburumieh, a fair-haired lady, is happy: Since I have been making a face pack with a mixture of 2 tablespoons of the miracle powder, 1 teaspoon of honey, 2 tablespoons of curd cheese and 1 yolk, my complexion is more tender and my skin smoother. Even the wrinkles disappeared. Margarete Aburumieh recommends: „Apply up to twice a week, depending on the type of the skin, 10 to 20 minutes this syrupy face pack, then rinse off with cold water."

Her husband, head physician Dr. Abdul Aburumieh, 40, in Melk an der Donau, takes the stone flour: „Already after ten days I felt more well-balanced." Now he checks, if the miracle powder reduces his elevated **colesterol level.** If this is the case, he wants to recommend the heeling magma from the heart of the earth. „Anyway, too many medicines are prescribed. And there is hardly one without side effects. The stone flour be a good alternative."

Other, but nevertheless equally astonishing effects from the miracle powder from Austria, were achieved by the family Thannhäuser. Father Alex (48) and son Markus (17) from Kicking near St. Pölten have been taking the powder since 23 February. Alex Thannhäuser: „I feel more vital, my stinging pain in my foot have disappeared." Son Markus: „After a week I was better able to be attentive at school." The pupil in a „Gymnasium" wanted to be sure, middle of March he stopped to take the miracle powdor for two weeks – immediately he felt lifeless and tired.

Four test persons who, up to now, had only good experience. They will be joined by ten mor who are chosen by the Austrian television. They shall swallow the powder under medical supervision for a period of one year.

„Die ganze Woche" reports 1986:

Cure Naturally: The Primary Rock Flow!

It is today „the talk of the town", this primary rock flow from the Waldviertel. A really impressive, constantly growing number of people who are looking for a cure, tell really wonderful stories about it.

Is all this really true, does its effect stem from a collective „autosuggestion?" Primary rock flow has been used for a long time for the improvement of the soil, to produce compost, and lately also to save the forests.

What seems to be new is that one can swallow it, without danger regularly, and thus alleviate or even cure diseases.

By no means! This method of treatment is not new, it has a tradition for thousands of years! From ancient time people used again and again certain healing minerals, healing loam or „healing earth", successfully as a remedy for external and internal application against **rheumatism** and **metabolic disturbancess**.

But how can one explain the effect of this mineral powder?

○ On the one hand because of its marked detoxicating effect: the fine powder can „bind" toxic substances in the intestines and thus make sure that they are excreted.

○ On the other hand by an – up to now unproved – absorption of mineral elements into the blood circulation and into the lymphatic system, so virtually, through a compensation of mineral defieiency symptoms. The mineral elements and the trace elements have for the organism an importance similar to that of the vitamins and the enzymes.

A further advantage of this remedy lies, no doubt, in the fact that very high temperatures are produced during grinding, and it thus becomes virtually free from germs.

Shall one take it or not – that is the question! Ask your family doctor and your reason, if there is anything that speaks against it – just like with any other medicine.

„Aargauer Woche" reports on 3 July 1986:

Now also in Kanton Aargau.
„Miracle Stone Flour" from Austria is very much in the News!

aw. The discovery of the veneer wood manufacturer Robert Schindele in the village Gansbach-Kicking in Lower Austria has, in the meantime, become known all over Europe: He wins from his quarry a stone flour, to which special effects are attributed. The small village, consisting of only a handful of houses has turned to a real „place of pilgrimage" for ill people.

This unbelievable story started with Schindele buying a large forest. He built forest roads for a better economic development and paved it with this crushed stone from his quarry. Instead of the sickening trees becoming sicker from this dust, the contrary happened: The trees became distinctly healthier.

„If this helps my woods, it will help me too", the resourceful Mr. Schindele said to himself. He ate some ground wake and it is said that since that time he feels much better, previous complaints are said to have disappeared. The news spread rapidly, and when the Austrian television transmitted a broadcast about the stone flour, the actual rush started. Among the people ordering is also King Fahd from Saudi Arabia. The Schindeles gave up their production of veneer wood, and since then they try to manage, to some extent, the flood of orders.

Schindele had his polygenous analyzed and the special composition with 21 minerals certified. Silicic acid, aluminium oxide, potassium oxide ferrous oxide make up the main components. He „baptised" his stone flour with the name „Superbiomin".

All over the world

Materials like silicic acid, potassium or iron have certainly been known in medical science for a long time. Uric acid has the reputation to keep young the **skin**, the **nails** and the **hair**. Potassium improves, as it is generally believed, the **supply of blood**. Especially women need to take a sufficient amount of iron which is very important for them.

The first customers of the stone flour were Austrians and people from Western Germany. Many of the tourists in Austria interrupted their leave for a few days, to get to Gansbach-Kicking. Every day the family Schindele receives up to 1500 letters. the telephone line is constantly busy. In the meantime the stone flour has been sold to all five continents – also to Switzerland and to the Aargau. Mr. Schindele is not afraid that the reserves could be exhausted soon. He estimates that the deposit consists of 2.5 million tons.

„St. Galler Nachrichten" report on 10 July 1986:

Health Through the Miraculous Stone Flour „Superbiomin"!

Robert Schindele (54) from Lower Austria was not very healthy and felt rather uneasy. Gouty pains troubled him: Severe pain! For twenty years he has been suffering from impaired digestion – spasms of the stomach troubled him and colics made his life difficult. When Robert Schindele celebrated his 50th birthday he had already snow-white hair.

Today everything is completely different. The **blood values of the Austrian are good, his gout** has disappeared. His **stomach and intestinal tract** are functioning perfectly, and – it is hardly believable – his previously white hair have partly turned black again!

The magic word is „Superbiomin". Robert Schindele eats every day one spoon of this wonder drug. This remedy is broken in the quarry. „Superbiomin" is simply wake, ground to powder! But certainly not any wake, but a sort of primary rock, similar to lava.

But what gave Schindele the idea to eat stones – even if they are in pulverized form? Everything started, when crushed stone was exploited from the quarry on the property of the wood manufacturer Schindele, which was used to build a street. The undergrowth of the adjacent woods, belonging to the forest owner Schindele was covered by white dust. Schindele's anger was replaced by joy, when a year later he noticed that his trees that had been damaged by the acid rain, seemed to have revived: they grew higher up, the needles grew darker, and finally new, healthy shoots developed. Robert Schindele conjectured and concluded: the stone powder apppears to be at the bottom of it.

A chemical analysis proved that he was right. The stone flour contains minerals that plants need urgently, minerals that are, in this composition also for human beings very useful. These are: silicic acid, potassium, calcium, iron, magnesium, zinc etc.

One can only confirm: this earth can work wonders. Every person who has swallowed the stone flour is said to feel much younger and more vital. It is said to help men against **disturbances of the potency**.

The minerals contained in the rock powder have a positive effect on the state of health:

Silicic acid is good for the **supply of blood**.

Potassium is effective against a **cardiac infarct**.

Chromium reduces the **blood pressure**, regulates the **colesterol level** of the blood and widens the blood vessels.

Magnesium supports the growth of the **cells**, calms the **nerves** and helps against **stress**.

When taking the stone flour „Superbiomin" from Robert Schindele from Lower Austria, the supply of practically all mineral elements is ensured, because the polygenous that is exploited in Mr. Schindele's quarry, then pulverized, contains many mineral elements and trace elements more than those identified by Dr. Schüssler at that time. Furthermore is should be pointed out that the stone flour of Mr. Schindele is a „purely biological product".

Bio-Mineral, Poststraße 14, St. Gallen
Telephone number: 233993.

A further press report:

New Remedy Discovered Against the Dying of the Woods?

By Rainer Rixen

He is sure to have discovered the philosopher's stone. Green, silvery, white, black lines, brown spots – the piece of stone Robert Schindele (53) holds in his hands shines in all colours. „With it we will save our forests! And our health!"

We travelled to the much-extolled Wachau in Austria, tosee in situ: What is this all about the wonder stone? Mr. Schindele discovered it; he maintains that this wacke – pulverized to powder – can save dying trees and cure human beings.

Looking down, the Danube is glittering below us. The first tourists sit outdoors, enjoying the sun and the juicy roast pork with „Waldviertler Knödel" (dumplings). Up here, 200 meters above the Danube, the wind caresses through the full crowns of the fir trees, the thrushes are twittering, the first broom blossoms.

The „miracle stone" lies below us, 20 millions of tons! Fire trees and spruce trees cover it. „For the time being I want to exploit 2.5 million tons" the man next to us, dressed in green, says. He wears a green suit in the style of a traditional costume, a green hat, he drives a green Mercedes 250 with a sticker on it saying, „wood has future".

The skilled charcoal burner, now dealer in wood and veneer wood manufacturer, bought five years ago a forest. „It looked quite bad. Many trees were sick. I had stones broken from a slope and the road fixed, so that, later on, we could better transport away the wood.

But then something surprising happened: „the fir trees at the roadside suddenly got new shoots, juicy and green. I pondered and concluded.

There was just one answer possible. My stone must have been for the trees like an elixir of life."

Schindele had his polygenous analyzed in Vienna by „ÖKO-Datenservice". It contained 21 minerals and metals. He told a medical doctor about this discovery. „This sounds like a wonder medicine" he said. Schindele took it verbally and in spoonfuls. Since that time my **gout** and my **colics** have disappeared!"

I take a few stones into my hands. They fall apart easily into layers. One can nibble them just like a piece of hard chocolate. It is, of course, easier with the powder, of which Mr. Schindele always has a sack full in the boot of his car. In the inn "Gasthof zum Schwarzen Bären" he takes a heaped tablespoon with two big beers, and drinks a glass of rosé wine afterwards. „Half a year ago I would have writhed with pain after that." I also try a spoonfull. It is like fine sand, without taste.

„Rock flow is nothing new and can definitely be effective" said Dr. Achim Dorenbusch (31) from the „Institut für Waldbau", University of Göttingen. „It is technically and economically a bit of a problem, because enourmous quantities are needed."

And what about health? „The stomach can absorb one or the other mineral or trace element that is good for the body", Dr. Josef Kiem (39), chief of the laboratory for trace elements research in the Kernforschungs-Institut Jülich, said. „Silicic acid (two thirds of the polygenous) is, for example, good for the intestines. The question is, if one can find in nature a mineral compositon that has the right dosage to eliminate deficiencies."

„Kremser Zeitung" reports in August 1986:

Mainly Germans Buy „Superbiomin".
„Miraculous Drug" from Kicking Still Sales Hit!

KICKING. – The sales boom of the stone flour exploited from the Jauerling and sold in Kicking (municipality of Dunkelsteinerwald) has been lasting already for several months.

The name of the miracle drug is „Superbiomin", it has been protected by patent, the name of its discoverer, Robert Schindele, has by now become known all over Europe. Already now, the sale of the „wonder drug" flourishes in the small, sleepy village. But as of this late autumn it will really start.

While the material is ground at present in a mill, according to instructions by Mr. Schindele, he wants to take over soon the whole production himself. At present a mill is built in Kicking. The project costs „several millions" (Schindele's daughter Edith), it could, if the demand for Biomin continues at this level, soon be amortized.

According to expertises, the stone flour from the Jauerling contains more than trace elements (minerals) and helps against practically all complaints. It helps against **metabolic disturbances, uric acid, colesterol** and **blood pressure disturbances** as well as against **weakness of the gums**, bad **digestion** and **thin hair**. It is said that the hair does not turn grey so fast . . .

Although since the beginning of the stone flour-boom every second car in Kicking has a German licence number, the success of the „miracle drug" stays at the moment within limits. Edith Schindele: „In Germany „Superbiomin" is now under the law governing the manufacture and prescription of medicines. It may be sold there only by medical doctors and in pharmacies." But, nevertheless, the weight bridge for the clearance of lorries, mainly for the export (most important market: Ferderal Republic of Germany) is going to be installed next to the mill.

It may be expected. Not even the consequences of the catastrophy of Tschernobyl could affect the sale of this remedy. And soon after the incident a certificate was available at Kicking that testified the harmlessness of the stone flour. Finally, nobody eats too much of this powder, which, even after hours, sticks in the teeth.

Martin Kalchhauser

„Apotheker" reports on 11 August 1986:

Test with Miracle Earth: Wrinkles Gone, Rheumatism Better

BILD der FRAU reported about the miracle earth, that is supposed to rejuvenate and make healthier – now Dr. Prinzenberg, a pharmacist from Bochum, made available the first results of success from patients:

○ A housewife (46) made face packs from the mineral powder, she says: „I now have less wrinkles."

○ A cashier (51) takes three teaspons full every day: „My **rheumatism** in my right hand has nearly disappeared."

Hair, skin, nails, Paramenia and buoyance are also influenced positively by the rock flow that contains minerals, Dr. Prinzenberg says. The miracle earth („Original Schindele's Mineralkur") can be bought in pharmacies and in health food shops.

„Die Welt" reports on 10 March 1987:

„Mineral Powder is not Harmful". – Import from Austria Prohibited due to Formal Reasons / Four Kilos for the White House!

Sabine Kobes, Bonn

In the Federal Republic of Germany the mineral flow from Lower Austria has been occupying the authorities and the courts of justice for months. Ronald Reagan did not seem to be influenced by this: It is said that four kilogrammes went to Washington a few weeks ago. The US President was very satisfied with the effect of the elixir, a representative of the White House wrote in a letter of thanks to the quarry owner Robert Schindele. This information we received from our Viennese correspondent Kurt Pollak. Since the summer of last year it is difficult for Germans to get the stone flour.

„I only have powder left for ten days, what shall I do after that? I do not want that my loss of hair and my backache return again . . ." Urgent calls for help, similar to this one, reach the 54 years old Mr. Schindele every day, since the import of his „Superbiomin" to the Federal Republic of Germany has been prohibited.

Five years ago he had a forest road covered with crushed stones, in order to be able to have his vehicles for the transportation of wood also go, even if rainy weather may come. Trees at the roadside that were dying, recovered within three months. The power of the stone flour, Mr. Schindele thought at that time, should also relieve human beings from their sufferings.

Since that time up to one hundred orders come in at Gansbach-Kicking every day. The family Schindele sends the powder in sealed tins as far as Australia. But since the time Mr. Schindele has a costant feud with the authorities concerning the import to Germany, some customers of „Superbiomin" became disconcerted.

The officials of the Ministry of Social Affairs of Hessen, who first had stopped the import, reassure that „Superbiomin" is, according tothe present knowledge, not at all harmful.

The reason for the prohibition were „of purely formal nature", Ministerialrat Albrecht Fuchs explained: „The way the manufacturer Schindele makes the advertising for his product, gives to the customer the impression that „Superbiomin" works as a medicine. But there was never placed an application at the „Bundesgesundheitsamt" (Federal Public Health Office) to have it registered as a medicine."

Schindele's reply to these remonstrances: „It is wrong to classify „Superbiomin" as a medicine. In actual fact it is a basic food that makes up the deficit of nutrive substances that are necessary for the energy balance of the human body." Each ton of the powder contains 128 kg magnesium and 140 kg potassium. It has a high content of silicic acid, aluminium, iron as well as of numerous trace elements. **Hypertension, arthrosis, scia-**

tica, disturbed circulation, gout and **rhumatism** can be combatted with the supply of minerals.

Mr. Schindele would not want to make use of the possibility to have his rejuvenating elixir registered as a medicine, if the German authorities insist on it: „In this case it could be sold in pharmacies and it would cost more than DM 3.50 per kilogramme, its present price", he says.

If you want to use the powder from the Wachau in Germany, you have to go over the border to the Netherlands, Belgium or to Switzerland, where you can buy „Superbiomin" without any problems. Other people buy the 40 kg-bags (Schindele: „This is sufficient for 20 years") directly in Lower Austria.

The „Hessische Verwaltungsgerichtshof" (Higher Administrative Court of Hessen) in Kassel will deal, probably during this month, with the protest of Mr. Schindele against the prohibition. The new mill, which the people from the Wachau have built at a cost of AS 20 millions, and which has been into operation at the end of last year, untiringly produces the beige powder with the worldwide protected name.

In the meantime Mr. Schindele has built a laboratory next to his quarry. Here scientists shall prove that those are right who regard the rock flow as a „gift from the Gods" or send to Mr. Schindele reports of success similar to the following: „My blood pressure went down. After that an acquaintance put some stone flour on the earth of his gum tree, and within 14 days it got seven new leafs. And his wife got rid of her rash."

„Kanada Kurier" reports an 28 May 1987:

Our Readers' Opinion.

Superbiomin

It is a miracle drug against **arthritis** and **bursitis**. Since it has helped so much my brother Henry Wittenberg, I then ordered one kilogramme for myself, because I too had arthritis in my right shoulder, so that I often could not sleep during the night. After having taken it for three months, my pain has disappeared, also if we have rainy weather which we often have her in B. C. I can sleep very well and work well in our flower garden. Our daughter had **bursitis** for six years and sometimes cried all night. She tried a lot of things, nothing helped her. Then she was operated, they took a small piece of bone out of her right shoulder, but it helped only for a short time and the pain increased. Our daughter-in-law who works as a nurse in the hospital, took her to a specialist for this disease. After he had examined her he told her she should not have been operated, because of this operation she lost the synovial fluid. He gave her an injection which released the pain for three months, she started again to work asa hair-dresser, but not for a long time, the pain came back. My brother and I advised her to take „Superbiomin", but she said she had tried somany things, she would wait. So I ordered one kilogramme of „Superbiomin" and had it sent to her, and after taking it for six weeks she said that her pain was easing off, she could sleep through, and after having taken it for four months she is healthy again, can use her right arm just like before, works again and has ordered already ten kilogrammes. Everything that she used to do for years with her left arm, also when driving a car, she now can do again with her right arm and use it fully.

We are thankful to God with all our heart, for the lovely nature with all its flowers, bushes and trees and also for the mountains, from which we can get the heeling remedy, for the people who produce „Superbiomin" of it.

A. Barger,
Abbotsford, B. C.

„Die ganze Woche" reports on 11 June 1987:

Heeling Earth and Primary Rock Flow!

Symptoms of mineral deficiencies have nowadays – mainly due to a wrong, too one-sided „sour food" – become more frequent than the often cited vitamin deficiencies.

But without sufficient supply of minerals also some vitamins do not work effectively.

These „trace elements" are important substances, that can be found in the organism in tiny little quantities, but that are of extreme importance for the whole metabolic process!

The most important mineral elements are: natrium, potassium, calcium, magnesium.

The most important trace elements are: iron, copper, zinc, selenium, cobalt, chromium, iodine, manganese, molybdenum, phosphorus etc.

But how to take it? The most extensive and most effective method has always been and is still today the intake of ground earth substances. Therefore also the name „heeling earth".

A few months ago some very contradictory rumours have been going around, that concerned more the activities of profiteers, but not necessarily the undisputed effectiveness of the method. There is no doubt that the regular intake of powdered minerals (as heeling earth or as rock flow) influences very positively the mineral metabolism of the human being – but also of the animals and the plants – and therefore can stop them!

„Frau und Freizeit" reports in July 1987:

Universal Remedy Stone Flour

Schindele's stone flour is again on the market. Although the first boom about the „Wonder Powder Superbiomin" has calmed down, there is still a great number of enthusiastic followers who have absolute confidence in it, now as ever.

Do you remember? About a year ago the press reported in quick succession virtual acclamations. „Wonder stone", „philosopher's stone", „30 years younger with 'Superbiomin'" was the tenor. The reason for this euphoria was the discovery of the 55 years old veneer wood manufacturer Robert Schindele from Kicking in Lower Austria, who, by chance, discovered the advantages of the said stone flour, as a „medicine for sick trees".

1000 GRAMMES SUPERBIOMIN CONTAIN:

SiO_2 silicic acid	622.000 g
SiO_3 silicic acid	11.617 g
Al_2O_2 aluminium oxide	183.300 g
K_2O potassium oxide	78.000 g
Fe_2O_3 ferrous oxide	48.000 g
CaO cacium oxide	11.000 g
MgO magnesium oxide	14.400 g
Na natrium	11.000 g
Mn manganese	0.350 g
Cu copper	0.061 g
Zn zinc	0.095 g
Co cobalt	0.019 g
Mo molybdenum	0.024 g
B boron	0.007 g
Ch chromium	0.029 g
N nickel	0.027 g
V vanadium	0.110 g
Ph phosphorus	0.058 g
N (Kl) nitrogen	0.113 g
N (tot) ammonia nitrogen	0.172 g
N (org) organic nitrogen	0.170 g
Rest trace elements and water	

„What helps the woods, may also help me", the man suffering from gout thought and started to swallow stones. Finely pulverized, of course, and after an analysis, that revealed respectable data. The wacke contains a lot of valuable minerals, mainly silicic acid, aluminium oxide, magnesium oxide and 18 other, vital substances.

Robert Schindele's state of health improved rapidly, his pain disappeared completely, the **loss of hair** was stopped, moreover, – in his snow-white hair some black strands grew again.

No wonder that Mr. Schindele thought to have found a universal remedy, which he made public and sold at a ridiculously low price. In the meantime thousands of people swallow his „Super-Biomin" and a flood of letters of thanks reach the „wonder quarry-owner". The diseases cured or at least improved reach from **rheumatism** to **migraine**, from **arthrosis** to **disturbed digestion**.

But also enemies ask for the floor, mainly from the circles of the classical medicine who call the stone flour simply a nonsense. On the other hand there are medical doctors who treated their patients successfully with „Super-Biomin", but can explain its effect only to a certain extent.

This is the reason why this product, after an absence of half a year, now again is available in pharmacies, but without the indication remedy.

There is no doubt about the effectiveness of the rock flow on the growth of plants. For the forest soil as well as for the garden mould, fertilization with „Super-Biomin" means an enrichment with minerals, which are often missing in the soil due to constant fertilization with chemical fertilizers. With it a better supply of nutrive substances is effected, chemical fertilization and the use of insecticides can be reduced to a great extent.

It is only logical that the mineral elements the plants are missing, also lack in our nourishment.

One thing is certainly clear: „If it does not help, itcertainly does not harm", „Super-Biomin" is nevertheless for many people a hope for recuperation they do not want to miss.

„Die Zeitung für den Konsumenten" 1987 reports:

Stone Flour „Superbiomin": How Mother Earth Takes Care of Us!

A year ago or two there was a lot of sensation about the „stone flour" from Lower Austria: old age symptoms are said to be combatted, grey hair turn dark again, and it can perform other miracles. Many people swear by it, others smile about the „superstition", television deals with it, and, last not least, the public health authority prohibited everything – anyone could come!

Actually, the agitation about the „wonderful stone flour" of Robert Schindele from Gansbach-Kicking only proved that nobody was really informed. For primary rock flows have been serving, since ancient times, often as the only (!) fertilizer for fields and meadows, e.g. mire of the NIle in Egypt or glacier water in Wallis, Switzerland. The action was recognized scientifically about the middle of last century and has been used since that time in the biological farming. Today one talks about „trace elements" the body needs just in tiny little quantities; without them nothing functions in a living organism!

Now, the trace elements all come from the bowels of the earth, from vulcanic primary rock", as e.g. granite, basalt or diabase. Under the influence of wind and weather rocks decay to pebble gravel, to sand and finally to fine dust or loam. The fertility of every tilled soil depends very much upon the wacke it is made from, because the plants dissolve with the acids of their roots the minerals and make use of them according to their needs. The trace elements then get via the vegetable food into the body of the human being and the animal.

Our digestive system works similar to the roots of the plants: if you swallow fine primary rock flow, parts of it is dissolved in the stomach and in the intestines and absorbed by the body. And since we have today a deficiency of one or the other trace element, the stone flour brings the missing elements, and „wonderful" effects result. But, if someone does not have any such deficiency, the stone flour does not bring him anything.

The mentioned stone flour „Schindele's Superbiomin" is now again available, it is to be taken with a liquid and does practically have no taste at all. The effect is the more convincing, the stronger a person suffers – for whatever reason – from the deficiency of trace elements. The proof of the pudding is in the eating! No risk, because undigested stone flour leaves the body without causing any complaints.

The pharmacist Magister Doskar, who took over the sale of Schindele's „Superbiomin" with firm conviction, stresses its very fine pulverization and especially the 20 elements in this „primary rock flow" that are soluble in gastric acid. Schindele's „Superbiomin" is sold in pharmacies and in chemist's shops.

Mr. Robert Schindele was internationally distinguished for „Superbiomin" with the following documents and medals.

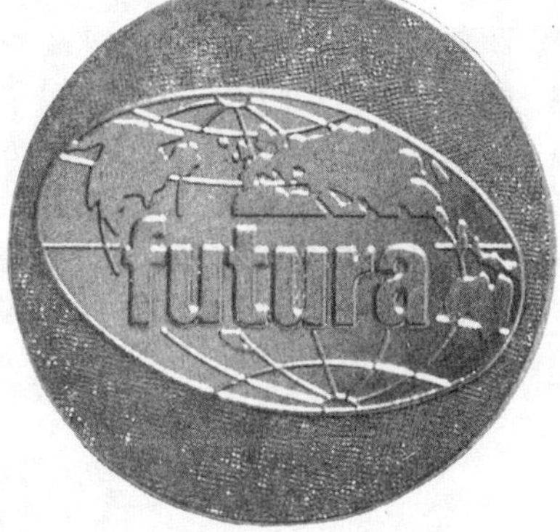

Futura 1986, Strasbourg

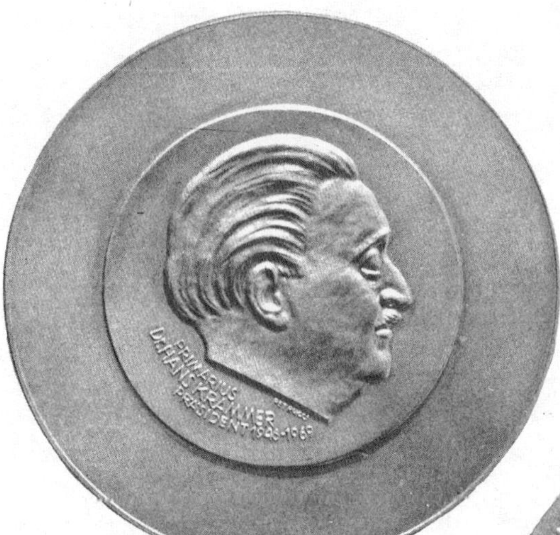

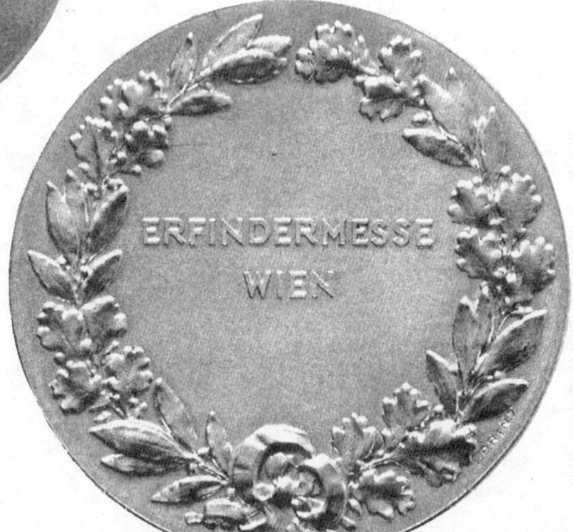

Österreichische
Erfindermesse, 1986

IENA 86
INTERNATIONALE AUSSTELLUNG "IDEEN-ERFINDUNGEN-NEUHEITEN" NÜRNBERG 1986

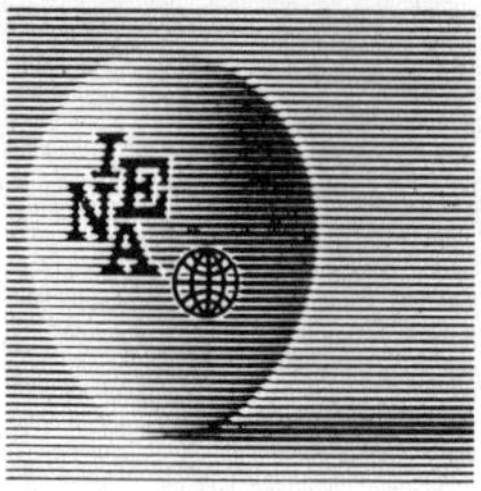

EHREN~URKUNDE

Robert Schindele, Österreich

wurde für hervorragende Leistungen

eine Silber-Medaille

verliehen

Erfindung/Neuheit: Flora Mineralsteinmehl

Nürnberg, 8. November 1986

Die internationale Jury der IENA 86

futura 86 STRASBOURG

PALAIS DE LA MUSIQUE ET DES CONGRES

DIPLÔME

MEDAILLE D'OR

décerné á Mr. Robert Schindele

pour URGESTEINSMEHL

PALAIS DES CONGRES futura STRASBOURG

AOUT
1986

La direction

URKUNDE

DER ÖSTERREICHISCHE PATENTINHABER- UND ERFINDERVERBAND

VERLEIHT

HERRN ROBERT S C H I N D E L E

FÜR

S U P E R B I O M I N

DIE

GROSSE MEDAILLE IN GOLD

DER PRÄSIDENT:

(Ing. Helmut JÖRG)

Wien, im September 1986

Epilogue

I have been working in the wood line of business for 41 years and since 1948 self-employed. I was for many years a member of the „Fachverband der Chemischen Industrie und des Holz- und Baustoffhandels" (trade association of the chemical industry and of the wood and building material business) and at present I am a member of the „Fachverband der Holzindustrie und der Stein- und Keramischen Industrie" (trade association of the wood industry and of the stone and ceramics industries). Furthermore, I am a member of the „Österreichisches Kuratorium zur Rettung des Waldes " (Austrian curatory for saving the woods); of the „Akademie für Umwelt und Energie" (academy for environment and energy) in Laxenburg-Vienna; of the „Österreichische Bodenkundliche Gesellschaft der Universität Wien" (Austrian society for soil science of Vienna University), and of the „Internationale Bodenkundliche Gesellschaft" (international society of soil science) in Wagensingen, Netherlands, from where I constantly get valuable information material. Furthermore, I own some large forest enterprises in different climatic zones.

Because of the sightworthy forest tending of my woods many international excursions come. For many years I have been dealing with forest genetics.

During the decades of observing, when buying veneer wood for my factory, which usually is done from the trunk and at all seasons of the year, and by my watching the processing, I succeeded in deciphering the genetic information code of some of the most important species of deciduous trees.

I can read from the leaves of e.g. more than one hundred oakwood trees like in an open book all characteristics of the woods (colour, direction of the grains, if a long or a short stem, hardness, speed of growth, development of branches and passive eyes etc.) in a few seconds.

Because of that I am and always was ahead of my competitors.

I succeeded also in constructing the largest wood stock of moorland oaktrees of the world (more than 4000 years old, on the outside already carbonaceous, oak trees).

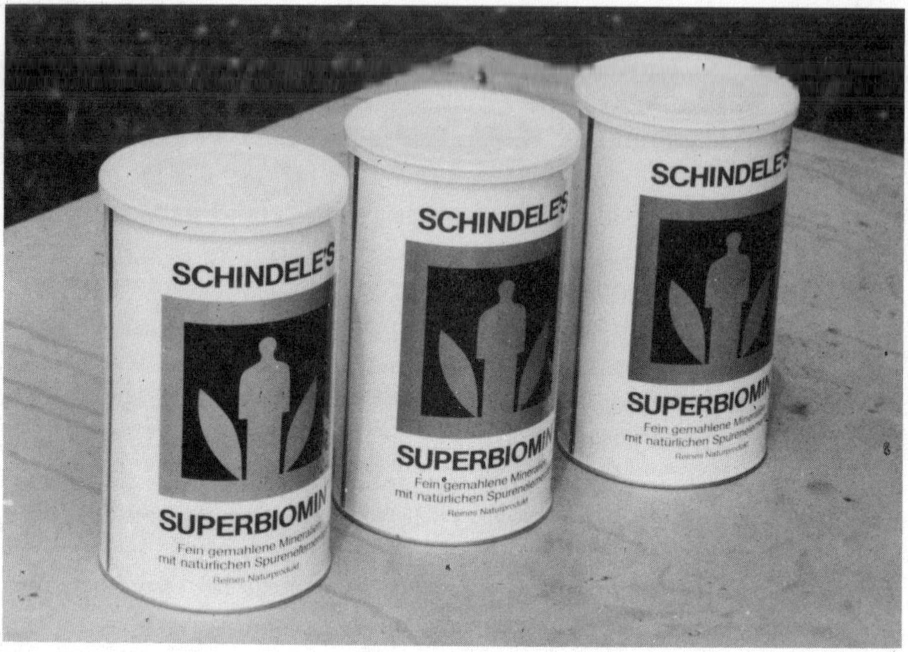

You can buy Superbiomin:

in all health food shops,
chemist's shops,
pharmacies
or directly from the manufacturer:

Mineralwerk Robert Schindele & Co. OHG.
A-3122 Gansbach Kicking
tel. no. 0 27 53 / 289

Index of illnesses